EDUCATED GUESSES

EDUCATED GUESSES

MAKING POLICY ABOUT MEDICAL SCREENING TESTS

Louise B. Russell

A Copublication with
the Milbank Memorial Fund

UNIVERSITY OF CALIFORNIA PRESS

Berkeley   Los Angeles   London

*A copublication with
the Milbank Memorial Fund*

University of California Press
Berkeley and Los Angeles, California

University of California Press, Ltd.
London, England

© 1994 by
The Regents of the University of California

Library of Congress Cataloging-in-Publication Data

Russell, Louise B.
    Educated guesses / making policy about medical
screening tests / Louise B. Russell.
        p. cm.
    "A copublication with the Milbank Memorial
Fund."
    Includes bibliographical references and index.
    ISBN 0-520-08365-2 (cloth : alk. paper).—
    ISBN 0-520-08366-0 (pbk. : alk. paper)
    1. Medical screening—Cost effectiveness.
2. Medical screening—Government policy—
United States. 3. Cervix uteri—Cancer—Diagnosis—
Cost effectiveness. 4. Prostate—Cancer—Diagnosis—
Cost effectiveness. 5. Hypercholesterolemia—
Diagnosis—Cost effectiveness. I. Milbank Memorial
Fund. II. Title.
    [DNLM: 1. Diagnostic Tests, Routine—utilization—
United States. 2. Predictive Value of Tests. 3. Preventive
Health Services—economics—United States. 4. Cervix
Neoplasms—diagnosis. 5. Prostatic Neoplasms—
diagnosis. 6. Hypercholesterolemia—diagnosis.
7. United States.   WP 480 R964e 1994]
    RA427.5.R87   1994
    362.1′77′0973—dc20
    DNLM/DLC
for Library of Congress   93-8768

Printed in the United States of America
1 2 3 4 5 6 7 8 9

The paper used in this publication meets the minimum
requirements of American National Standard for
Information Sciences—Permanence of Paper for Printed
Library Materials, ANSI Z39.48-1984. ∞

For Bob and Ben

Contents

List of Tables
and Figures

Tables

Figures

Foreword

The Milbank Memorial Fund is an endowed private operating foundation that has contributed since 1905 to innovation in health and social policy. The Fund's partnership in publishing with the University of California Press exemplifies its mission of using fresh ideas and information to improve health policy, especially in the broad areas of prevention and the allocation of resources.

Louise Russell describes how this book was written and reviewed in her Acknowledgments. The Fund assisted her in testing her ideas and analyses with decisionmakers in the public and private sectors as well as with scholars, scientists, and physicians. Our assistance was possible only because the extraordinary people whose names she lists share the goals of the Fund.

Russell is as extraordinary as any of the colleagues she thanks. For many years she has proposed and defended conclusions that are thoroughly grounded in research but are, nevertheless, disconcerting to many people. Intervening to detect or prevent disease is not, she has insisted, always a better choice than inaction. We are grateful to her, and to the people she cites, for their contribution to public understanding of the complexities and opportunities of health policy.

Samuel L. Milbank   Daniel M. Fox
Chairman   President

Acknowledgments

The Milbank Memorial Fund supported the writing of this book, but its president, Daniel M. Fox, did much more than that. It was his idea that a book should be written and that it should grow out of the Fund's Policy Review on Prevention. As part of this review an expert advisory group and invited guests met several times to discuss issues not only for the book but also for a television documentary on prevention being produced by Roger Weisberg of WNET-13 in New York. All but one of the meetings were held before I began to draft the manuscript. The people who attended brought with them an enormous wealth of information, experience, and wisdom from which to draw ideas for the book. Developing the book in this way was an exhilarating experience, quite unlike the slower and more uncertain process by which my earlier books, written without such distinguished help, had begun. I am grateful to the Milbank Fund, and to Dan Fox, for thinking of book writing in such unusual terms.

The advisory, or core, group for the project was made up of Kathleen S. Andersen, senior program officer of the Milbank Fund, Ronald Bayer, Dan Fox, Larry O. Gostin, Robert S. Lawrence, Jane Sisk, Thomas Vernon, Roger Weisberg, and me. This group met in August 1991 to decide on a framework for the meetings to follow and to discuss some early ideas for the book and the documentary. Bob Lawrence's remarks about screening at this meeting were particularly influential in my thinking.

In September, members of the advisory group met with Roger Herdman, Alan Hinman, Marshall McBean, and Deborah Stone for a day-long discussion that ranged over a variety of issues having to do with public and private roles in prevention. The November meeting focused on screening, and the advisory group was joined by David Eddy, Susan Gleason, Paul Griner, and David Naylor. The effects of lifestyle on health was the subject of the February meeting, at which the advisory group was joined by Warren S. Browner, Richard Daynard, Paul Fischer, Martin Redish, and Ernst L. Wynder. All of these individuals contributed to the yeasty atmosphere in which my ideas for the book grew. Dan Fox's summary remarks at the September meeting suggested the title and gave me the overarching theme for the book.

Several other people were especially helpful during the preparation of this volume. Linda Johnson White of the American College of Physicians brought me up to date on the college's work on common screening tests. Michelle Brattain researched the many newspaper and magazine articles on screening that help to set the stage in each chapter. William C. Taylor, who introduced me to the cholesterol controversy years ago and has kept me supplied with the latest medical literature, continued to keep me up to date as I wrote and revised the chapter on cholesterol screening.

I served as a member of the U.S. Preventive Services Task Force, chaired by Bob Lawrence, and of the Institute of Medicine's Committee on Clinical Practice Guidelines, headed by Jerome Grossman. The education I received while on both committees provided an essential foundation for writing the book.

Many people reviewed the first draft of the book and provided helpful comments: Warren Browner, Gordon DeFriese, Daniel Fox, Alan Garber, Paul Griner, Lee Greenfield, David Mechanic, David Naylor, Charlene Rydell, Jane Sisk, Michael Stapley, Barbara Stocking, Bill Taylor, Thomas Vernon, and Roger Weisberg. My colleague at the Institute for Health, Health Care Policy, and Aging Research, Gerald N. Grob, read parts of the manuscript in draft form and provided editorial comments.

Kathleen Andersen and Harriet Katz, with help from Daniel Klein, worked with me and Roger Weisberg on the logistics of the meetings.

Marilyn Schwartz guided the manuscript through the publication process at the University of California Press. Julie Carlson edited the manuscript, Catherine Sexton designed the figures, and Marcia Meldrum prepared the index. I am grateful to them for helping make the book clearer and easier to read and use.

All of these people have contributed to the finished product that follows. The responsibility for the opinions expressed and for any errors remains mine.

Louise B. Russell
Rutgers University
New Brunswick, New Jersey
August 1993

1

Introduction

Medical screening tests are familiar to nearly everyone, thanks to magazine and newspaper articles, programs on radio and television, and the literature in doctors' waiting rooms. All these sources report the advice of medical experts about who should get the tests and when—tests for high blood pressure, for high cholesterol, for diabetes, for breast cancer, colorectal cancer, and other cancers, for osteoporosis, for glaucoma. The list goes on and on. Not many people in the United States get through life these days without knowing about, and being subjected to, several of these tests, usually more than once.

The point of each test is to detect the condition before it produces symptoms. A common theme runs through the articles, programs, and waiting-room brochures: catch it early, treat it early, and live longer. If the condition is not fatal, the promise of longer life is replaced with the promise of pain and disability prevented by early detection. The test is usually quick, easy, painless or almost so, and, of course, worthwhile because of the ill health—not to mention the disruption and expense—avoided by acting before the disease becomes serious. And if the test turns out to be negative, the reassurance is worth the minor inconvenience.

That common theme, played out in its many variations, is simple, direct, and misleading. The straightforward recommendations about screening tests and the information that usually accompanies them are pseudo-truths. They convey rules of thumb developed by experts and leave out the complexities and tradeoffs, the mixture of solid information and educated guesses, that have gone into their development. Like the pseudo-elements of the physical sciences that bear a deceptively close resemblance to the real thing, the pseudo-truths about screening tests are not what they appear to be.

The term *pseudo-truth* would be unfair if the complexities and tradeoffs were not important or if the choices made by the experts were those the doctors and patients who use the tests—and the employers and taxpayers who pay for them—would make themselves with the same information. But that is often not the case. This book examines the complexities and tradeoffs involved in screening for three conditions—cervical cancer, prostate cancer, and high cholesterol—to show that the experts' recommendations are far simpler and more solid-looking than the evidence behind them. The recommendations are built on major decisions about what is worthwhile, for whom, and when. Sometimes the fuller truth bears only a superficial resemblance to the confident exhortations.

The pseudo-truths matter because they affect so many people and so much of medicine. Screening tests are pervasive. They constitute, or lead to procedures that constitute, a large part of medical practice. When the U.S. Preventive Services Task Force developed guidelines for clinicians, forty-seven of the sixty groups of preventive services the task force reviewed were composed of screening tests, with several tests—the major ones used to screen for a particular condition—included in each group.[1] Many of the tests are recommended for a large part or all of the adult population. Some are recommended for children as well. The growth in screening tests has been enormous in recent years. Familiar examples make the point: screening for high blood pressure became recommended practice only about twenty years ago, screening for high blood cholesterol less than a decade ago, and new tests are developed every year.

It is important to think about policy toward this large and growing aggregation of services. The experts' recommendations do not offer many choices, but the fuller truth does, and those choices should be made well because they involve the lives and resources of millions of people. Patients, clinicians, and payers need to recognize the extent to which the guidelines gloss over or ignore considerations of potentially great importance to them. For patients, the questions have to do with whether a screening test is the best way to spend time, emotional energy, and money to preserve or improve personal health. For doctors and their professional associations, the questions center on the most productive way to spend the ten or fifteen minutes allotted to each patient's appointment and, of course, the impact of the answers on their professional lives. For payers, the issues have to do with how best to spend employers' or taxpayers' money to improve health—or even whether the money would be better spent in alterative ways. Policymakers whose responsibilities extend beyond screening or medical care know that these alternatives are not abstract ideas; they involve real people with genuine needs and concerns who can be vigorous in the advocacy of those needs and concerns.

The screening tests discussed in this book were chosen with the advice of an expert group convened by the Milbank Memorial Fund. In four day-long meetings, these experts and their invited guests offered a wide range of ideas and information that helped shape this book. The tests discussed in the following chapters were chosen not only because they are important in their own right but also because they provide good examples of problems and issues that apply to screening tests more generally.

Chapter 2, on cervical cancer, serves as a textbook example of effective screening. Since the effectiveness of the Pap smear is well established, it is possible to focus on the surprisingly complex choices that remain, particularly the large personal and resource costs involved in such decisions as how often to have the test. The complexities arise from the nature of cervical cancer, the costs of screening and follow-up, and the fact that all tests are wrong some of the time—they miss some cases of disease and incorrectly identify other people as having the disease when they do not. As a result, the health and dollar costs of too much screening are large. They should be weighed against the costs of too little screening when recommendations are being formulated, but in the United States they seldom are.

Chapters 3 and 4, which deal with screening for prostate cancer and high blood cholesterol, bring out even more fundamental issues. By itself, even the most accurate screening accomplishes nothing. If it is to be effective, it must meet two more requirements: there must be effective treatment for the condition, and treatment must be more effective when delivered early, before the disease becomes obvious through symptoms. If either requirement is missing, screening contributes nothing to better health. The cases of prostate cancer and high blood cholesterol show that even for widely accepted and frequently used tests evidence that their use is effective is often simply not there. Screening for both conditions is recommended as much out of hope as on the basis of scientific fact.

The final chapter draws conclusions for the three examples and for screening tests in general. It raises questions about how tests are evaluated, recommendations are formed, and medical resources are allocated. In doing so, it stresses, as the earlier chapters do, the full range of consequences—the benefits and the costs, both personal and national. The chapter points out the opportunity costs of current recommendations, that is, the benefits lost when one possibility is put aside in favor of another. These benefits—what could be gained if things were done differently—are the true cost of decisions made about screening tests.

Some of the conclusions will be considered controversial and upsetting by many in public health and medicine. Individual screening recommendations are sometimes defended on the ground that even if the test itself is not useful, it serves an important purpose by bringing the patient to the doctor's office when nothing else would, thus giving the doctor the chance to evaluate the patient's health and needs more generally. The concern and caring for patients that underly this argument are praiseworthy, but the argument itself is at odds with the principle that modern medicine should be scientifically based. Science requires that services be proven beneficial by solid evidence. It is not enough that some experts believe they are beneficial. Medical care is only justified when it makes a difference to people's health.

This book is motivated by the belief that resources for medical care should be allocated so that they do as much as possible to improve the life and health of the population. To meet this goal, allocation decisions must be based on the best scientific evidence about what works, for whom, and at what cost. The United States spends vast sums on medical care, more than any other industrialized nation, and screening drives a large share of this expenditure. Thus understanding the full range of choices offered by screening tests is a critical starting point for understanding how to make the medical system serve the nation better.

2

Screening for Cervical Cancer

The Papanicolaou test for cancer of the cervix has been advocated for use as a screening tool since the 1940s.[1] Today it is an established, widely used test that is often the main reason a woman visits her doctor regularly. The test consists of scraping cells from the cervix, the neck of the uterus, onto a glass slide.[2] The smear is then sent to a laboratory where it is stained and examined under a microscope for evidence of abnormal cells, and a report is sent back to the doctor describing the findings.

Part of the truth, the well-known part, is that the Pap test detects precursors of cervical cancer as well as cancer itself, and that early detection and treatment reduce the death rate from cervical cancer to substantially below what it would be without screening. In the original Papanicolaou nomenclature, the precursor stages are described in order of severity as mild, moderate, or severe dysplasia. These are followed by localized cancer of the surface tissue lining the cervix, called carcinoma in situ, and finally by invasive cervical cancer. In recent years other classification systems have been proposed, all based on the idea of steady progression from early, easily treated abnormalities to cancer.[3]

Early abnormalities can be followed up and treated with relatively simple outpatient procedures.[4] Depending on the first report, an abnormal Pap smear may be followed by a repeat smear a few months later, or by colposcopy, a procedure for viewing the cervix under magnification to identify the size and location of the abnormality. Colposcopy is often accompanied by the taking of a tissue sample, or biopsy, to test further for cancer. A condition short of invasive cancer may be treated by freezing, cautery, or laser to remove the affected tissue, or, when the abnormality is judged to be too extensive for such methods, by cone biopsy or hysterectomy. Cone biopsy, removal of a section of the cervix, and hysterectomy, removal of the entire uterus, require hospitalization. Invasive cancer is treated by hysterectomy, or, if the cancer is advanced, by radiation.

Early treatment usually means that the condition never progresses to invasive cancer, so it is both more effective and less traumatic than treatment at a later stage. A landmark study conducted by the International Agency for Research on Cancer (IARC) shows that screening and early treatment can reduce the incidence of cervical cancer by more than 90 percent.[5] The study, vastly larger than any that preceded it, analyzed data for 1.5 million women screened over many years in eight countries to determine the impact of different screening schedules.[6]

Many women probably remember that the standard advice used to be to get a Pap smear every year. Indeed, they may not be aware that the standard has changed, since many physicians still advocate annual tests. But in 1980 the American Cancer Society came out with a new recommendation indicating that, if the first two annual tests were negative, subsequent tests could be given every three years.[7] For the next several years, the major professional organizations with an

interest in the Pap smear engaged each other in a vigorous
debate. The result was a consensus recommendation published in 1988 stating that women should receive Pap smears
as soon as they became sexually active, and no later than age
eighteen, and that tests should be given annually for at least
three years. If all of the first three tests are negative, subsequent tests can be scheduled less frequently at the doctor's
discretion.[8]

That the major professional organizations changed their
earlier clear and simple recommendation to a more complicated one, leaving the exact frequency of the test in the hands
of the doctor, suggests either that something changed or that
the underlying situation had always involved more complica-
tions. The new element was that careful estimates had
been made of the costs and benefits of different screening
schedules.[9] But the underlying situation had always been
more complicated, as suggested by the fact that some industrialized countries had screened less often than annually for
years.[10] The estimates served to make aspects of that complex-
ity explicit.

Accuracy of the Test: Missing Disease

No test separates those who have the disease from
those who do not with perfect accuracy, and the Pap smear is
no exception. In fact, there has been concern in the last few
years that, in the United States, the Pap smear is substantially
less accurate than it can or should be. Stories in major newspapers and magazines have emphasized the frequency with
which cases of cervical cancer are missed. Most report that 15
to 20 percent of cases are missed at a single screening, and the
number may be as high as 45 percent.[11] The IARC study found

that some countries with centrally organized screening programs served by one laboratory had achieved considerably greater accuracy, with an average of only 6 to 7 percent of cancers missed at one screening.[12]

There are three reasons why a cancer might be missed—two of them avoidable. The first is that the scraping of cervical tissue taken by the doctor may not include abnormal cells, even though abnormal cells are present elsewhere in the cervix. This is particularly likely to be the case when cells have not been taken from the endocervix, or transition zone, the area where abnormal changes usually show up first.[13] The second reason is that, in examining the hundreds of thousands of cells on a slide, the lab technologist may miss the few abnormal ones. The third reason is that cancer develops after one test and sometimes progresses far enough to produce symptoms before the next one. Most cervical cancers develop slowly, taking an average of eight years to progress from a detectable abnormality to invasive cancer, and thus regular tests will detect them in an early stage.[14] But a few develop more quickly, producing symptoms before the next test is due.

To counter the substantial risk that a cancer will be missed, a woman usually has only one option presented to her—to have the test more often.[15] If the errors are independent—that is, if there is no reason to believe that an incorrect reading on one test increases the chances of an incorrect reading on the next—two tests will be much more accurate than one.[16] For example, when the error rate of the test is 20 percent, twenty of one hundred women with cervical abnormalities will be missed by the first test and eighty will be correctly diagnosed. When the twenty women whose abnormalities were missed appear for their next test, the probabilities will be the same—20 percent (four women) will be missed again, and 80 percent (sixteen women) will be correctly diagnosed. Thus, after two tests, only four of the original one hundred cases will not have been detected. After three tests, only one will still be undiagnosed.[17]

Some clinicians urge testing annually or even every six months exactly for this reason, especially for high-risk women.[18] Since most women have at least one risk factor, these exhortations come close to the old recommendation of annual tests for everyone.[19] Factors that are believed to put a woman at higher risk for cervical cancer include smoking, being sexually active as a teenager, having more than two sexual partners in a lifetime, having a partner who has had several partners, having several children, and using oral contraceptives.[20] More recently, infection with the human papilloma virus has been associated with a greater risk of cervical cancer.

A woman might consider the time, inconvenience, and cost well worth the extra margin of safety, particularly given that, as an individual, she has so few options for influencing the accuracy of the test. Stories in the major magazines and newspapers adopt this point of view, citing the rate of missed cancers and showcasing the tragic or near-tragic consequences for individuals. An article in the *New York Times Magazine* ends on this note: "In general, the gynecologists' advice boils down to this: when in doubt, have a Pap test every year. 'To do any less,' says Dr. George W. Morley, of the University of Michigan Medical Center, 'is to play Russian roulette with your life.' "[21]

Accuracy of the Test: False Positives

Not one of the stories mentions that, like all tests, the Pap test is subject to another kind of error—it classifies women as having precursor conditions when, in fact, they do not. The problem is that the precursors are not clearly distinct from other abnormal states. Common conditions like inflammation or injury to the cervix produce tissue so similar in appearance to dysplastic tissue that they can lead to a mistaken diagnosis when the sample is examined.[22]

Over the course of her lifetime, a woman is more likely to have a Pap test that *incorrectly* identifies her as having a condition that might develop into cervical cancer than she is to develop cervical cancer.[23] Studies indicate that the Pap test probably produces incorrect positive results more than 1 percent but less than 10 percent of the time.[24] If it does so 5 percent of the time, then in the course of having ten tests a woman has a 40 percent chance of at least one false positive (Table 1). If each of one hundred women undergoes ten tests, forty of them can expect to be incorrectly diagnosed as having a precursor to cervical cancer by at least one of those tests.

In spite of the fact that the rate of false positives is only on the order of 5 percent, false positives occur much more often than missed cases of cancer because *all* women can experience a false positive. Only those who actually develop cervical cancer can experience a false negative. Without screening, the chance of developing invasive cervical cancer is 2.5 percent for the average woman over her lifetime and the chance of dying from it is 1.2 percent.[25] Thus, at most, two or three of every one hundred women will eventually develop a cervical cancer that could be missed by the test, while all one hundred are vulnerable to the possibility of a false positive result.

The more often a woman has the test, the higher the probability that she will have a false positive. If the false positive rate is 5 percent for one test, the chance of having at least one false positive is 40 percent for ten tests, 54 percent for fifteen tests, and 64 percent for twenty tests (Table 1). A woman who

Table 1   Probability of at Least One False Positive Test
(as a percent)

Number of Tests	Probability if the False Positive Rate for One Test is	
	5 Percent	0.5 Percent
10	40.1%	4.9%
15	53.7	7.2
20	64.2	9.5

NOTE: The calculations apply to an individual woman who undergoes 10, 15, or 20 tests, but it is easier to explain them in terms of the results for 100 women. If the false positive rate for one test is 5 percent, 5 of the 100 will experience a false positive on the first test, 95 will not. At the second test, 5 percent of the 95 who have not already had a false positive (4.75) will experience a false positive (as will 5 percent of the 5 who have, 0.25), so that the total number of women with at least one false positive after two tests is 9.75 (5 on the first test and 4.75 on the second). For one woman, this means that her probability of a false positive after two tests is .0975 (9.75 divided by 100).

The calculations proceed in the same manner for subsequent tests. At the third test, 90.25 women still have not had a false positive and 5 percent of them (4.51) will, raising the total to 14.26, and so on through the total number of 10, 15, or 20 tests. The calculations are made on the assumption that the chance of a false positive on each test is independent, that is, a false positive on one test does not mean that the woman has a greater (or smaller) probability of a false positive on the next test.

conscientiously goes in for yearly tests starting at age eighteen will have more than fifty tests in her lifetime. Increasing the frequency of the test increases one type of error while reducing the other.

The only way to reduce both errors—false negatives and false positives—at the same time is to improve the quality of the test in the first place, through more complete tissue scrapings and more accurate readings. Table 1 shows the much lower probabilities of at least one false positive if the rate for a single test is only 0.5 percent, which is at the extreme of the estimates of accuracy published in the medical literature. Even then, a woman is four times as likely to have at least one false positive over the course of twenty tests as she is to develop cancer in her lifetime.[26]

In weighing the risk of missing a cancer against that of a falsely positive test, women should keep in mind that false positives lead to further diagnostic tests and, often, to treatment. Rather than take the chance of ignoring a true precursor condition, the physician may proceed with treatment, with its risks, pain, and costs in time and money. The risks include hemorrhage, infection, and unnecessary hysterectomy.[27] False positives also engender worry and stress since the woman herself has no way to know that she does not have cancer or a precursor. When the test result is incorrect, these risks and costs are undertaken without any benefit to the woman. Doctors, on the other hand, do well by doing good— testing more often and following up conscientiously to be sure that no cancer is missed while collecting more fees for the additional work.[28]

Even when the test correctly identifies a precursor, early treatment may be wasted because the condition would never have developed into cancer. The so-called precursor conditions do not inevitably progress toward cancer; often they revert to normal. This may be one of the areas of knowledge about cervical cancer that is most uncertain, and, with Pap screening so common, it will not be easy to determine the facts. One review of the evidence concludes that perhaps one-third of cases of mild and moderate dysplasia do not progress to a more serious stage and might revert to normal, and that even carcinoma in situ often improves without treatment rather than advancing to invasive cancer.[29] The currently accepted view is that both failure to progress and reversion to normal are most common in women under forty or fifty years of age.[30]

The Benefits of Screening

The benefits of screening for cervical cancer are conventionally measured in terms of cases of disease prevented and lives extended—when cancer is prevented, some women live longer. Data from the IARC study show that screening every ten years reduced the number of cases of invasive cervical cancer by two-thirds (Table 2). Because earlier abnormalities were detected and treated, the cancers simply never got started, or never progressed to the invasive stage. The number of cases was reduced by more than 80 percent when screening

Table 2   Reduction in Cases of Invasive Cervical Cancer Achieved by Different Frequencies of Screening

Years between Tests	Reduction (%)	Number of Tests
10	64.1	3
5	83.6	6
3	90.8	10
2	92.5	15
1	93.5	30

NOTE: Based on screening women once before the age of 35, again at 35, and then at the frequency shown until age 64, when screening is discontinued.

SOURCE: IARC Working Group on Evaluation of Cervical Cancer Screening Programmes, "Screening for Squamous Cervical Cancer: Duration of Low Risk after Negative Results of Cervical Cytology and Its Implication for Screening Policies," *British Medical Journal* 293 (September 13, 1986): 659–64.

took place every five years. Annual screening brought the reduction to almost 94 percent. The primary gain comes from instituting any sort of regular screening schedule—even every five or ten years. More frequent tests bring smaller additional gains.

Since only about half of women who get cervical cancer die of it, not all of the prevented cases contribute to longer life. Eddy has developed a mathematical model to translate the IARC data into days of life and has used it to examine the effect of screening at intervals of four years (a frequency not reported in the IARC study), three years, two years, and annually. Compared with no screening at all, screening every four years from age twenty to age seventy-five was estimated to increase the average woman's life expectancy by about ninety-four days, or approximately three months.[31] The gain appears relatively small because the large benefits for those few women who are spared cervical cancer are spread over all women screened. (Recall that average does not mean low-risk. The factors believed to increase the risk of cervical cancer are so widespread that the average woman will have at least one.)

Increasing the frequency of screening by one year is estimated to add about 1.5 days of life per woman—for example, screening every three years increases life expectancy about 1.5 days over screening every four years, screening every two years adds another 1.5 days compared with screening every three years, and annual screening adds still another 1.5 days over screening every two years. Each increase brings some benefit, but the additional benefit is much smaller than the gain that comes from the initial introduction of screening. False positives and the natural regression of precursor states have little effect on these calculations because follow-up and treatment rarely cause death.

If benefits were measured in terms that included the quality of life, false positives and regression would play a larger part. More women undergo the stress, discomfort, and risks of treatment needlessly than undergo them with benefit—recall the lifetime probabilities of a false positive as compared with cervical cancer itself. Adding the possibility that a correctly identified condition would never have progressed to cancer, especially in younger women, increases the number of cases in which treatment provides no benefit.

As the IARC data suggest, the greatest impact on health can be achieved by screening women who are not being screened at all, or not with any reasonable regularity.[32] The model estimates that screening a woman who has never been screened saves about sixty days of life, compared with the three days saved by screening a regularly screened woman once a year rather than every three years. The large majority of women in the United States report having had a Pap test in the last three years, according to a national survey done in 1987, but approximately one-quarter have not (Fig. 1). Young women were the most likely to have been screened. Older women and women of Hispanic origin were the least likely.

The Costs

The issue of first importance for any medical intervention is its impact on health. Although there are many uncertainties about the Pap test and about cervical cancer, the evidence strongly supports the conclusion that screening for cervical cancer lengthens lives. Its effect on the quality of life, through the impact of false positives and the unnecessary care that accompanies them, has received less attention. Unless women place no value on quality of life, which seems unlikely,

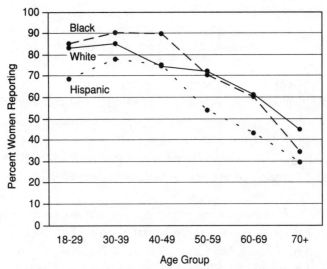

Figure 1. Women Reporting Pap Smear within Last Three Years: United States.
Notes: Based on a sample of 12,599 women. Women who had never heard of the test—2.1% of whites, 4.1% of blacks, and 15.1% of Hispanics—were omitted, as were the 3.6% of all women who could not remember the date of their last test. *Source:* Linda C. Harlan, Amy B. Bernstein, and Larry G. Kessler, "Cervical Cancer Screening: Who Is Not Screened and Why?" *American Journal of Public Health* 81 (July 1991): 886.

an assessment of the benefits of screening should include these effects as well as gains in length of life.

Once the benefits of an intervention are established, the costs of achieving those benefits need to be considered. Women, physicians, and policymakers measure costs differently because of their different situations. If the woman has a good medical insurance plan, at least for follow-up procedures if not for the test itself, neither she nor her doctor may consider cost an issue because the major portion will be paid by the plan. If she does not, they may have to. From the larger perspective of the nation, however, costs cannot be ignored. Whoever writes the check, the Pap test and the follow-up procedures must be paid for with funds that could have been used to meet other needs—needs that will remain unmet if the resources are claimed by screening for cervical cancer.

An obvious part of the costs of screening for cervical cancer is the Pap test itself. At a cost of $75 for the test and the visit to the doctor, it has been estimated that screening every adult woman in the United States between the ages of twenty and seventy-four every three years would cost about $2 billion a year.[33] Screening every year would cost about $6 billion annually.

By itself, however, screening does no more than identify women who might benefit from further care. The full costs of screening include the costs of the follow-up and treatment necessary to make a difference to health. Conservative follow-up of mild or moderate dysplasia costs between $50 and $70.[34] More aggressive follow-up might include surgery to remove abnormal tissue. If no abnormality is found, some physicians proceed to cone biopsy rather than take the chance that the abnormality is simply difficult to find by current diagnostic methods. Costs of treatment can range from $300 to $1,300. While early detection saves some money, since the precursor stages are not only more effectively but more inexpensively treated than later stages, the saving only partly offsets the costs of the test and of treating false positives and conditions that would have regressed on their own. The offset is smaller the more often the test is performed because of the burden of false-positive results.

When the costs of screening and follow-up are compared with the gains in days of life, what benefit is purchased at what cost? To answer this question, Eddy applied the same model he used to estimate days of life saved.[35] Figure 2 shows the cost of saving a year of life by different schedules—screening every four years, every three, every two, and annually—compared with no screening at all.[36] Screening every four

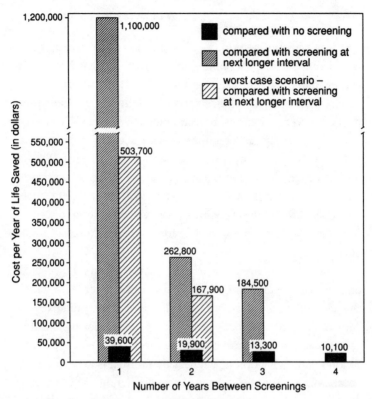

Figure 2. Cost per Year of Life Saved for Different Frequencies of Screening
Notes: Future life-years and costs (in 1985 dollars) are discounted at 5% per year. All assumptions are based on data for an average woman who is asymptomatic when she begins screening at age 20 and who is screened to age 74 or 75. *Source:* David M. Eddy, "Screening for Cervical Cancer," *Annals of Internal Medicine* 113 (August 1, 1990): 218, 222.

years saves a year of life for about $10,000, screening every three years costs $13,300 per life-year, and even annual screening costs only $39,600 for each year of life saved. These costs are in line with those of other widely used medical interventions, such as drug treatment for high blood pressure or bypass surgery.[37]

Screening at some frequency is thus a reasonable investment by current standards, but which frequency? That depends in part on the additional cost required to save an additional year of life by screening more often—every three years rather than every four, say, or annually rather than every two. The results show that once screening is more frequent than every five years, increasing frequency is an expensive way to extend lives (Fig. 2). Compared with screening every four years, screening every three costs an additional $185,000 for each life-year saved. Increasing frequency from three years to two brings additional life-years at a cost of $263,000 each. And compared with screening every two years, annual screening costs more than $1 million for each additional life-year saved.

Some experts are concerned that the nature of cervical cancer may be changing, so that past experience—on which the estimates are necessarily built—is a poor guide to the future. They believe that cervical cancer is increasing and that fast-growing cancers are becoming more common, especially among younger women. There is by no means agreement on these points. One study showed that screening itself, which is sought more often by younger women, could create the illusion that fast-growing cancers are more common.[38] Another found no evidence for more rapid-growing tumors in younger women in Australia, where the concern has also been raised.[39]

Figure 2 shows results for a "worst-case" scenario based on a series of assumptions that reflect these concerns. The worst case assumes that invasive cancers occur at three times the rates observed in the United States in the 1980s, that the rate is higher than in the past for women ages fifteen to twenty-four, that fully one-fifth of abnormalities are of a type that progresses to invasive cancer in less than two years, and that the Pap smear is 15 percent more likely to miss a cancer than in the IARC study. (These results can also be viewed as representing the situation for women who are at higher-than-average risk.)

This combination of dire assumptions makes surprisingly little difference to the general conclusion that increasing frequency is expensive. Compared with no screening, screening every three years costs $15,500 per life-year, somewhat more than before, because the lower accuracy of the test and the greater number of rapidly growing tumors mean that more cancers are missed, but not a great many more. Increasing the frequency of the test to every two years costs an additional $168,000 for each additional year of life (Fig. 2). And compared with screening every two years, annual screening saves extra life-years at a cost of more than $500,000 each.

Because they are based on data from the IARC study, the estimates in Figure 2 reflect the high accuracy of the test in countries with centralized screening programs. Both the rate of missed cancers (3 percent) and the rate of false positive results (0.5 percent) for a single round of testing are much better than the rates thought to be true in the United States. As already discussed, lower accuracy gives both women and their doctors reason to test more often in order to increase their chances of correctly detecting a cancer before it has progressed too far. At the same time, more frequent testing greatly increases the burden imposed by false positive results. Thus inaccurate tests create two costs—the resource cost of doing the test more often and of the associated follow-up and treatment, and the cost in personal suffering of women who go through follow-up and treatment needlessly. From the policymaker's point of view, more frequent testing is questionable medicine and an expensive way to compensate for inaccurate tests. If annual testing costs $6 billion and triennial testing costs $2 billion a year, several billion dollars a year could be spent on improving the quality of the test and everybody would be better off.

At the same time, there are many women who are not tested frequently enough by any standard. For these women, testing can be cost-saving. A study of low-income elderly women who had not been screened in many years, if ever, found that a single screening saved money and extended lives by detecting conditions that would otherwise have been very expensive to treat, or too far advanced to treat successfully.[40]

A Textbook Case

Screening for cervical cancer provides a particularly good example of the elements involved in any screening intervention because its effectiveness is well established, and thus the issues are not confused by doubts about whether it works. Effectiveness depends on a continuous chain that has no weak or missing links. There must be a stage before symptoms develop during which the disease, or its precursor, is detectable. There must be a test that can detect it with reasonable accuracy. And there must be treatment that, if delivered early, leads to better results than waiting until symptoms develop. For cervical cancer, these conditions are met.

Screening for cervical cancer demonstrates that, even when the facts are reasonably clear, a number of important and difficult decisions remain. Substantial effort has gone into quantifying the gains in length of life from the Pap smear and the costs of using it—work that raises critical questions about the almost automatic tendency to recommend that any effective test, especially if it is easy to administer, be done yearly. The resource costs of that automatic recommendation can be high and the benefits low. Yet even these complex analyses have not incorporated into their calculations the considerable burden imposed by false positives—a burden that continues to play little or no part in screening policy in the United States. False positives are particularly troublesome for a relatively rare disease like cervical cancer, because they occur much more often than the disease.

In contrast, cases of missed disease have played an important role in policy decisions, but with no more attempt to analyze alternative policies or quantify their consequences than in the case of false positives. Many physicians and their professional organizations continue to favor annual testing to offset the poor record of U.S. labs in detecting cancers. The costs of that policy, in resources and, because of the greater number of false positive results, in human suffering, have not been considered nor has the policy been compared with approaches that would act more directly to improve the accuracy of the test.

Medical policy at all levels—patient, clinician, interested professional societies and advisory groups, and insurers who pay for the test—has focused on the women who already come to the doctor's office and the frequency with which they should be screened. Little has been done to address the one-quarter of all women in the United States who are not screened even every three years. The gains in health from screening these women are much greater than the gains possible from screening the remaining 75 percent every year rather than every two or three years. The saving from less frequent screening of those already in the system would be enough to pay for the additional women and for a good deal else besides.

This contrast between the unserved 25 percent and the rest shows that it is possible to overinvest in an intervention and underinvest at the same time. For women who are screened regularly, increasing the frequency of testing from every two years to annually brings an additional year of life at the high cost of more than $1 million and an uncounted number of false positives. By contrast, for elderly minority women who have not been screened in recent memory, if ever, a Pap test can be cost-saving as well as life-saving.

There is, of course, no one technically right policy toward screening for cervical cancer, but not all scientifically based policies are equally good. Policies that miss many women entirely while spending lavishly on others bear rethinking. A better policy would consider all women and weigh not just gains in length of life, but improvements or declines in quality of life and the resources taken from other, possibly more beneficial, medical care. Ellman observes that recommendations must explicitly balance "the small but very serious risk of invasive cancer" against "the disadvantages of over-treatment." For the Pap smear—and for any effective test—"just as it is unethical to neglect the needs of patients, so it is unethical to squander resources and unethical to entangle patients in needless investigations and treatments."[41]

3

Screening for Prostate Cancer

The American Cancer Society recommends that all men over age forty get a digital rectal examination every year for prostate cancer. The exam is medicine at its simplest—the physician inserts a finger in the patient's rectum and feels, or "palpates," the back and sides of the prostate, a small gland that surrounds the urethra (the tube that empties the bladder) and that produces some of the fluid for ejaculation. If the physician detects irregularities in the prostate, he or she will recommend an ultrasound examination and, if necessary, a biopsy. Ultrasound provides a picture of the irregular area, but cannot show definitively whether it is cancerous or benign. When there is doubt, and with the ultrasound image as a guide, tissue samples are taken and examined to determine whether cancer is present.

The recommendation for annual exams appears routinely in newspaper and magazine articles about prostate cancer, along with some standard statistics about how often the disease strikes. One man in eleven will get prostate cancer, according to the statistics. It is the second leading cause of cancer in men. In any given year more than 100,000 men will be diagnosed as having it, and about 30,000 will die of it; for

1992 the estimates were 132,000 cases diagnosed and 34,000 deaths.[1]

The treatment for prostate cancer often causes impotence and incontinence. These side effects are so serious, and occur so frequently, that some writers of popular magazine articles spend considerable time discussing the recent advances that have made them less frequent, to reassure men that the treatment is not worse than the disease.[2] The goal of the annual rectal exam is, of course, to find the cancer early. If it is still contained within the prostate, surgery to remove the prostate is often recommended. In the past the procedure, called radical prostatectomy, virtually always caused impotence, and caused partial or complete incontinence in 16 percent of cases as well.[3] A modified procedure, introduced in the early 1980s, leaves intact the nerve bundles that control erection. About 35 percent of patients who undergo the modified procedure become impotent, and 5 percent suffer some degree of incontinence. Radiation is an alternative to surgery, but it too can cause impotence or incontinence.[4]

Side effects like these are enough to give a man pause as he considers whether to follow the American Cancer Society's advice. To encourage him the articles stress that the disease is most curable when it is detected early and that many deaths would be prevented if men would have regular checkups. A recent article in *Business Week* provides some persuasive statistics: "If the disease is discovered early, before it can spread, treatment is so effective that nearly 90% of all patients live at least five more years. And for all cases combined, the survival rate has increased to nearly 75% from 50% three decades ago. 'With those kinds of results, today's high mortality rate is just unacceptable,' says Curtis Mettlin, who heads an ACS [American Cancer Society] committee on ways to increase early detection of the disease."[5]

As further encouragement, a 1991 article in the *New England Journal of Medicine* reported that a blood test, prostate-specific antigen (PSA), in conjunction with a digital rectal exam, can detect more cancers than the digital exam alone, and at an earlier stage in the cancer's development.[6] The news was quickly picked up by the press, along with the lead author's recommendation that all men over fifty should have the blood test annually.[7]

Thus it appears that, thanks to scientific progress, the disease can be detected earlier, when the prospect for cure is best, and the cure is not as fearful as it used to be. Still, even with the new surgical procedure, a substantial number of men are left with impotence and some degree of incontinence. The situation is full of complexities and tradeoffs, more than enough, it would seem, to qualify it as the full truth about prostate cancer. And yet it is not.

But Does It Work?

Rarely does a news story mention that there is no evidence that going in for regular exams and pursuing treatment if cancer is found (with all its potential side effects) will extend a man's life. Indeed, there is some evidence that they will not. The knowledge is so common among urologists and other experts in the field, and the controversy over its implications so pervasive, that the fact does surface in an occasional story, but it is quickly countered in the same story by statements from other physicians that "logic tells you"[8] that early detection and treatment work, or that "you've got to be irrational"[9] to believe that they do not.

Yet the U.S. Preventive Services Task Force, an expert panel convened by the U.S. Department of Health and

Human Services to develop a guide for primary-care clinicians, wrote in its report that "the major randomized controlled trial comparing treatment of prostate cancer with no
treatment found that radical prostatectomy was no better
than placebo in altering five-year survival."[10] Another study of
U.S. patients, reported in the leading British medical journal,
the *Lancet*, found no evidence that regular digital exams
helped prevent metastatic prostate cancer, that is, no evidence that it caught cancers early enough to prevent their
spread.[11] Current therapy is largely ineffective once the cancer
has metastasized.

On its face, it sounds ridiculous to say that early detection
and treatment might not be beneficial. As one urologist, a
critic of screening puts it, "A fundamental principle of all
cancer management is that early detection offers the best
chance for cure."[12] Besides, there are those impressive statistics: When the disease is discovered early, almost 90 percent
of patients live at least five years; and the overall survival rate
has risen from 50 to 75 percent over the last three decades.
With numbers like that, how can it *not* be the case that screening and treatment for prostate cancer help men live longer?

The answer lies in the nature of prostate cancer and the
pitfalls of evaluating screening tests. Virtually all prostate cancer is found in men over fifty years of age—less than 1 percent
of cases are diagnosed in younger men.[13] Autopsy studies have
shown that as many as 30 percent of men between the ages of
fifty and seventy have evidence of prostate cancer; by the time
men are in their eighties and nineties, the percentages may be
much higher.[14] In the medical literature, the 30 percent figure
is accepted as a reasonable approximation for all men over
fifty.[15] These men died of other causes and, while alive, were
never diagnosed as having prostate cancer.

Thus there is a large reservoir of prostate cancer that is

never diagnosed *and does not need to be* because it never causes significant symptoms, let alone death. This pool of occult disease offers many pitfalls for evaluating whether screening and treatment help men live longer.

Evaluating Screening Tests

The first pitfall arises from the basic purpose of screening—to find disease early, when it is hoped that treatment is most effective. Survival figures, like the ones given in the *Business Week* article, measure the length of time a person survives after the disease is diagnosed, so they are affected by whether the diagnosis is made early or late in the course of the disease. For example, without screening, a man might be fated to discover that he has prostate cancer at age sixty-five, because of symptoms, and to die of it at age sixty-nine, four years later. With screening, the cancer might be discovered earlier, perhaps at age sixty-two. Even if treatment were no more effective at that point and the man still died of cancer at sixty-nine, the measured length of survival from the time of diagnosis would be seven years compared with four.

Survival statistics are usually reported in terms of the percentages of people who survive a certain length of time—five, ten, or fifteen years. In this case, the man would be counted a success if he were screened since he survived more than five years after diagnosis, but as a failure if he were not, since in that case he survived only four years after diagnosis. Yet either way he died at age sixty-nine. Indeed, the man was probably made worse off by screening because he suffered with the knowledge that he had cancer, and with the treatment and its side effects, for three years longer than if he had not been screened. This problem is known as "lead-time" bias, lead

time being the extra time added to survival after diagnosis by
the fact that the diagnosis was made early. The bias favors
screening, and because of it comparisons of survival times for
people who were screened and those who were not can be
misleading.[16]

A second problem arises from the fact that prostate cancers, like other types of cancer, are a heterogeneous lot—
some grow relatively quickly, others so slowly that they never
cause clinical symptoms, and still others fall in between. Slow-
growing cancers are more likely to be picked up by screening
because they are around longer in a presymptomatic state. A
slow-growing cancer might exist for two, five, or even ten
years in a state in which it caused no symptoms but could be
detected by a screening test. A fast-growing cancer might
grow from undetectably small to large enough to cause symptoms in less than a year so that even annual screening would
miss it—it would be too small at the first test, and would
already have become apparent before the next test was scheduled.

The consequence of this second kind of bias, "length" bias,
is that cancers discovered by screening are more likely to be
slow-growing ones with little or no impact on life expectancy,
while those missed by screening are more likely to be fast-
growing cancers that can shorten a man's life substantially.
Once again, when people whose cancers were discovered by
screening are compared with those whose cancers were not,
screening can look good even when it makes no difference.
This bias affects both survival times and statistics on the stage
of detected cancers. Staging statistics report the percentages
of cancers discovered in early and later stages, and a higher
percentage of early cancers is taken as a sign that screening
works. Slow-growing cancers are obviously more likely to be
discovered in an early stage.

A third potentially important bias in the case of prostate cancer is the bias from "over-diagnosis" or "over-detection." The point of screening is to discover potentially fatal cancers early enough to prevent death, but it can also discover cancers that would never have killed, or even produced symptoms. These cancers will make survival and staging statistics look good because they will generally be small and in an early stage and the men with them will live just as long as they would have without screening. In the case of prostate cancer, there is a large number of such cases that could be uncovered by screening. Again, comparisons with groups who were not screened will be biased because the cancers discovered in the unscreened group will be only those that caused symptoms, and they are much more likely to be cancers that also shorten life.

If the course of prostate cancer were perfectly understood, if the proportions of cancers of different types and the length of time each existed in various stages were known, it might be possible to correct for all these biases, but it is not. Only a randomized controlled trial can provide an accurate picture of whether screening and the treatment that follows discovery of a cancer actually help men live longer.[17]

The Gold Standard: Randomized Controlled Trials

A randomized controlled trial of screening must have at least two separate groups of people: one group is screened and the other is not. It may have more groups if there are several variations of screening—different tests or combinations of tests, for example—that need to be evaluated, but there must be a control group that is not screened, or not screened to as high a standard. In the latter case, the control group often receives what is termed "community care," that is, they and their usual doctors do whatever they would ordinarily do. The groups in which screening is being tested are given the best, state-of-the-art screening and treatment as defined by the physicians conducting the trial.

The second and even more critical feature of a randomized controlled trial is that the people in the trial must be randomly assigned to the screened or the control group. Assignment cannot be influenced by any characteristic of the person—such as age, risk factors for cancer, area of the country, or physician. Only if assignment is random can the evaluators be reasonably sure that the screened and control groups will be as alike as possible in every characteristic, those known and those not yet known to influence prostate cancer. And only if the two groups are as alike as possible can any differences in outcomes at the end of the trial be ascribed to screening.

The outcome measured by the trial—the "endpoint"—must be whether the person died from the cancer by the end of the trial. Even in a properly randomized controlled trial, endpoints short of death, such as survival from the time of diagnosis, are subject to the biases already discussed. But if significantly fewer people have died in the screened group by the end of the trial, that is solid evidence that screening works.[18]

Ideally a trial should be "double-blind," that is, neither the people in the trial nor the clinicians screening and treating them should have any idea who is in which group. The reason for this is that people sometimes see what they want to see rather than what is, and if they know which group is which, their beliefs may influence their reporting and thus the results of the study. Generally, a perfect double-blind is not possible in screening trials, but some parts of it can be protected from this bias. For example, the staging of cancers can be done by people who do not know whether the patient or tissue specimen before them belongs to the screened or the unscreened group.

No randomized controlled trial of screening has been done for prostate cancer.[19] The evidence that is available comes from uncontrolled studies. Thus it is impossible to know whether that evidence shows real benefit from screening and the subsequent treatment or is no more than the natural result of all the biases to which screening studies are subject. Randomized controlled trials are sometimes impossible to do when, even though there is substantial disagreement over the value of a medical intervention, experts think it would be unethical not to provide it. In the case of screening for prostate cancer, the differences in opinion are so great that a trial is considered justified and the National Cancer Institute has recently initiated plans for one.

The Prostate, Lung, Colorectal, and Ovarian Cancer Screening Trial includes prostate cancer along with several other cancer sites and will enroll 74,000 men (and 74,000 women) ages sixty to seventy-four.[20] The purpose is to find out whether screening can reduce the death rate from these cancers. After an initial examination, half of the men (and half of the women) will be screened annually for three years. The outcomes for both the screened and the unscreened groups will be followed for more than ten years; from start to finish the trial will take sixteen years. The large numbers and long period of time are necessary if enough deaths are to occur to show clearly which group does better. With good luck, the trial will provide a definitive answer to whether screening for prostate cancer extends lives. With bad luck, the trial may be so contaminated by uncontrollable influences from outside— if, say, men in the control group, affected perhaps by medical news and trends in the country at large, begin going to their own doctors for frequent screening—that the results will be suspect in spite of the most careful design.

The only randomized controlled trial that has been done for prostate cancer was of treatment, not screening: radical prostatectomy in the treatment of early-stage cancers. When the results for the men who were operated on were compared with those for men who received an inert pill, the investigators found no difference in survival at five or fifteen years.[21] With a total of only 111 patients in the surgery and control groups, the trial was not large enough to constitute strong evidence, but the results are not encouraging since they suggest that, even if screening successfully identifies the right tumors, the available treatment may not make a difference.[22]

Accuracy of the Tests

In the absence of good information about the effectiveness of screening and treatment, much of the debate has centered on the characteristics of the available screening tests, especially their accuracy. Just as with cervical cancer, a good test should be able to detect prostate cancer without missing many cases and without producing large numbers of falsely positive results. Current thinking, based on the idea that radical prostatectomy, or perhaps something else, will eventually be shown to reduce mortality, and the certainty that current treatment is unable to extend life once the cancer has spread, is that the test must not only detect cancer, but must detect it while it is still contained within the prostate. Biopsy, in which a sample of tissue is taken and examined for cancer cells, is used to follow up suspicious results and is the standard by which other tests are measured.

None of the tests is very accurate. The studies that have produced the best results are not applicable to the routine screening of healthy men because they were done with men who had symptoms suggesting cancer. Partly because of differences like these in the men studied, findings differ widely from one study to another. In addition, nearly all of the studies were conducted by urologists engaged in research; thus the screening was done by experts with particular interest and training in getting the best results. Mass screening, which would involve many nonspecialists, could be expected to be less accurate.[23] Three tests are the main contenders for routine screening: digital rectal exam; ultrasound imaging of the prostate; and the blood test for prostate-specific antigen (PSA).

The digital rectal exam is the oldest and most widely used of the screening tests. Its accuracy is inherently limited because the physician cannot reach parts of the prostate gland. Studies of men with symptoms suggest that the digital exam is capable of detecting as many as 70 to 80 percent of cancers. A study of men without symptoms, more typical of those who would undergo routine screening, reported that the rectal exam detected only 33 percent of cancers, missing the majority.[24] Unfortunately, the cancers are often found too late. About half of tumors thought to be confined to the prostate on digital examination are found to have spread when surgery is performed.[25] The exam produces many false positives—22 to 34 percent of positive tests turn out to be cancer when a biopsy is performed, while two-thirds or more are falsely positive.[26]

Transrectal ultrasound is a more recent test with the potential to detect smaller cancers, including cancers that are too small to produce a palpable irregularity in the prostate. Studies have shown that it detects from 21 to 91 percent of can-

cers, although, again, many of the studies involved men who
had symptoms or who were known to have cancer.[27] Like the
digital exam, ultrasound has a high yield of false positives,
partly because the images produced by cancers and by various
benign inflammatory conditions are so similar. Only 17 to 41
percent of positive tests are shown by biopsy to be cancer; 59
to 83 percent are false positives.

The digital exam and ultrasound are both invasive, and
their accuracy depends on the skill of the operator in using
and interpreting the technique.[28] The PSA test has attracted
interest because it is a simple, noninvasive blood test. The
test measures the level of prostate-specific antigen, an en-
zyme produced only by prostatic tissue.[29] The level increases
when cancer is present. For the version of the test approved
for use in humans in the United States, levels of 4 micrograms per liter (µg per liter) or higher are considered suspicious.[30] PSA was discovered in 1971 and is used to monitor
the effects of treating prostate cancer; it is considered "an
exquisitely sensitive tumor marker."[31] Its use in screening
asymptomatic men for prostate cancer is more recent and
more controversial.

Like the other tests, the PSA test fails to pick up many cases
of cancer and is elevated in many men who do not have
cancer. Thirty to forty percent of men with cancer confined to
the prostate have PSA levels of less than 4 µg per liter,[32] while
large numbers of men without cancer have elevated levels. In
particular, men with enlarged prostates, a very common condition in older men, have elevated PSA levels about one-quarter of the time.[33] The result is that PSA too produces a large
number of false positives—more than half of all positive tests
are not confirmed by biopsy.

Because each of the tests alone is so inaccurate, most clinicians believe that a combination of tests may be superior. The

widely reported article on PSA for screening used such a combination.[34] The PSA test was administered first. If two tests administered a week or two apart were 4 µg per liter or higher, a digital exam and ultrasound were performed. If they were normal, and the PSA level was less than 10 µg per liter, nothing more was done. If either showed abnormalities, or if the PSA level was 10 or higher, a biopsy was performed. The authors of the study reported that, of the 112 men who had biopsies, 37, or 33 percent, turned out to have cancer. The combination of tests did find some additional cancers, but, like each test alone, it also produced a large number of false positives—two-thirds of the men with suspicious findings on earlier tests had negative biopsies.[35]

The Current Situation

In the face of such low accuracy, and the lack of evidence that it is worthwhile to screen, some advisory groups have recommended against screening efforts. The U.S. Preventive Services Task Force stated that there was no reason to do rectal exams if a physician was not already doing them, although it did not go so far as to recommend that physicians who were already doing them should stop. The group recommended against the use of other tests for routine screening.[36] The Canadian task force recommended against any routine screening for prostate cancer.

At the same time, the American Cancer Society and the National Cancer Institute support the recommendation for annual digital exams, and stories in major newspapers and magazines regularly pass on this advice along with recommendations by individual physicians for the use of PSA or ultrasound. Real costs, in human suffering and in resources, are created by these recommendations, costs that will continue and probably even grow while further evidence is being gathered. It is important to be aware of those costs in considering the best policy to pursue until the effectiveness of screening is determined.[37]

The consequences of falsely positive test results are one of the costs, just as for the Pap smear. Most of the usual kind of false positives—men who test positive even though they do not have cancer—will be resolved by biopsy. Because each test has a large number of false positives, many men will be referred for a biopsy and most will not have cancer. The procedure is invasive and, depending on how it is done, may require the administration of antibiotics to reduce the chance of infection, and sometimes general anesthesia. Most patients notice some blood in their urine for a while after the procedure. According to one expert, the complication rate is 2 percent, "mostly minor."[38]

More frequent tests are another consequence of false positives. Once a man has had a positive test, even though it is not confirmed, his physician may want to check him more often. In the study of PSA as an initial screen, men who had negative biopsies were retested every six months, twice as often as men whose PSA tests were negative.[39]

A second sort of "false positive" for which the consequences will often be more severe occurs when cancer is discovered that, without screening, would not have surfaced during the man's lifetime. Here the test is correct in the sense that cancer exists, but there would be no point in treating it even if effective treatment were available. Aware of this, many clinicians are willing simply to monitor a small cancer in an elderly man, reasoning that he will probably die of other causes before it produces problems.[40] But for younger men, aggressive treatment is usually recommended. Thus a man whose cancer might never have amounted to anything faces the prospect of a 1 to 2 percent chance of dying during the surgery, and a one-third chance of impotence after it. One physician recommends that, until screening and treatment are shown to be effective, men should be presented with the current evidence and left to make their own decisions about whether they want to be screened.[41]

Many men will find themselves in the position of discovering silent cancer whether they choose to or not. Enlargement of the prostate is a common condition in men over age fifty and in about 15 to 20 percent the symptoms—difficult or painful urination—become severe enough to warrant surgery to remove part of the prostate.[42] Prostatectomies for the relief of prostate enlargement are one of the most common surgical procedures in the United States, and over 300,000 operations are performed each year.[43] When the surgically removed tissue is examined in the lab, 10 percent of the men—potentially over 30,000 a year—are discovered to have some traces of cancer.[44] In six of every ten cases discovered this way, the traces are so small that the physician may decide to do nothing but continue to monitor the case. In the other four, treatment will be recommended.

Thus the human costs of the current approach to prostate cancer include the potential for harm without benefit to several groups of men: men whose cancers are discovered and treated when, without screening, the cancers would have remained silent; men whose cancers are discovered as the result of surgery for an enlarged prostate but would not have surfaced otherwise; and false positives—men who undergo ultrasound and biopsy, but are not diagnosed as having cancer. If men in either of the first two groups are *not* treated, because their cancers are judged unlikely to progress during their lifetimes, they suffer the anxiety of having a cancer diagnosis and probably the inconvenience and discomfort of more frequent tests. Those who *are* treated suffer the often serious side effects of that treatment without any prospect of benefit. The false positives in the last group—an inevitable cost of any screening test—would, if screening for prostate cancer were effective, influence its frequency and the groups targeted. If screening is not effective, they are a cost with no compensating benefit.

The resource costs of screening for prostate cancer encompass the costs of the test or tests, physicians' fees, follow-up of positive tests, and any treatment recommended as a result of the tests.[45] How much is actually spent currently in the United States is not known, but it is clearly well below what it could be: survey data for 1987 show that no more than 20 percent of men get digital rectal examinations as often as the American Cancer Society recommends.[46] Because of the recent enthusiasm for the PSA test, which is more acceptable to patients than the rectal exam, the number of men who are screened regularly has probably increased since that year, but is still relatively low.

If all men were actually screened every year, costs would increase substantially. Men over age fifty would be screened at least once a year (interestingly, in spite of the American Cancer Society's recommendation, experts in the medical literature never suggest screening men under fifty). Estimates made in the late 1980s put the costs of screening alone, without the costs of the subsequent treatment, between $2 billion and $23 billion per year, depending on the screening tests and the cost per test.[47] The PSA test was not considered a useful screen at the time these estimates were made. A conservative estimate of the cost of screening with the digital rectal exam and the PSA test together, based on data for the late 1980s and early 1990s, is about $4 billion per year.[48] Like the earlier estimates, this one omits the costs of treatment and would be much higher if those costs were included.

An important question hangs over these estimates. Are the resources, and the pain of the men who are screened and treated, accomplishing anything? For the Pap smear, whose effectiveness is well established, the issues concern the right balance among missed cancers, false positive results, and resource costs. For prostate cancer the issue of balance may be meaningless since it has not yet been shown that the costs are counterbalanced by any benefits. The policy question for individual men, clinicians, and policymakers is what to do during the years it will take for definitive evidence to be collected.

Screening is valueless if no effective treatment exists. As noted earlier, one physician has recommended that men should be informed of the current situation and left to make their own decisions about whether to be screened. Unless their personal doctors agree with this view, however, many men will not know that there is a decision to make—they will simply accept their doctors' recommendation for screening and for any subsequent treatment. The man who is informed of the situation will have to decide whether he would prefer to accept screening and treatment, with all its disadvantages, or to take his chances with the cancer. The widely accepted public image of cancer as a relentless killer inclines many men to choose treatment, even when the doctor would prefer to wait.

The question came up on a larger scale in September 1992 when a drug company sponsored free screening for prostate cancer at two thousand medical centers across the United States. Critics charged that the free screenings were "little more than publicity stunts and money makers for participating centers, bringing thousands of men in for follow-up tests, biopsies and treatment that [might] not benefit them." A

supporter countered that he "would rather be unnecessarily
cured of a disease than fail to be cured of a disease that could
be the cause of my death."[49] Thoughtful observers, and patients, might well wonder what sense it makes to screen for a
condition when there may be no useful treatment for it.

Appendix: Details of the Estimate of Screening Costs

The estimate of screening costs is based on the assumption that all men will comply with the recommendations
for initial tests and any follow-up tests (100 percent compliance). The screening protocol is an adaptation of the one used
in the study by Catalona and colleagues.[50] In that study two
PSA tests were administered to each man a week or two apart.
If both were 4 micrograms per liter or higher, the man was
called in for a digital exam and ultrasound.

For routine screening it seems likely that if a man comes in
for a blood test, he will be given a digital exam at the same
visit rather than called for a second visit when the blood test
is positive. In fact, this is the procedure that will be followed
in the National Cancer Institute trial. If either the (single) PSA
test or the digital exam is positive, ultrasound will be recommended. In the study by Catalona and colleagues, about 5
percent of men referred for ultrasound were not biopsied
because the digital and ultrasound exams were normal and
the PSA, although elevated, was below 10 µg per liter. Because the percentage is so small, it has been assumed for this
estimate that all men referred for ultrasound are also biopsied.

The estimate is first calculated for a cohort of 1,000 men
fifty or older. The average cost per man is then applied to the

population of men fifty or older in the United States. The cost of the initial visit, with a digital rectal exam, is assumed to be $50 and the cost of the PSA test is also assumed to be $50.[51]

Cost of initial screening: 1,000 men × $100 = $100,000

In their study, Catalona and colleagues found that 8.3 percent of the men initially screened had elevated PSA values. If a digital exam were done at the same time, some men with normal PSA values would have suspicious findings from the digital exam. Chadwick and colleagues, who used both tests, reported that 20 percent of the men referred for ultrasound were referred on the basis of a positive digital exam alone. Thus the figure of 8.3 percent has been increased by 20 percent, to 10 percent, and 100 men out of the cohort of 1,000 would be referred for ultrasound and biopsy. Lee and colleagues put the cost of an ultrasound exam with biopsy at $350.[52]

Cost of follow-up ultrasound and biopsy:
100 men × $350 = $35,000

Catalona and colleagues found cancer in one-third of the men referred for ultrasound and biopsy. Their referrals were based on the PSA test alone, but, as reported in Chapter 3, one-third is also a reasonable estimate for the proportion of positive digital exams confirmed by biopsy. Thus 67 of the men referred would not be found to have cancer. They would probably be retested more frequently; in the study by Catalona and colleagues, men with negative biopsies were retested every six months. Thus these men would have a second series of tests in the same year as their first screening. The cost of this second screening is assumed to be the average cost of the initial screening, or $135. This underestimates the cost because it implicitly assumes that these men are no more likely than the average man to have abnormal findings on a second exam.

Cost of six-month retest: 67 men × $135 = $9,045

Adding these figures gives the total annual costs of screening for 1,000 men: $144,045. The average cost per man is $144. Except for the cost of the PSA test, the costs per visit and procedure are from the late 1980s, and may have been low even for that period.

If all of the 28 million men fifty or older in the United States were screened according to this protocol, the total cost would be just over $4 billion per year. If, in addition, the 15.5 million men ages forty to forty-nine were screened, the cost would be substantially higher. An estimate has not been made of the additional amount, however, because there are no studies on which to base estimates of the numbers of men in this age group who would be referred for ultrasound and biopsy.

4

Screening for High
Blood Cholesterol

A randomized controlled trial is the strictest scientific test of whether screening or other medical interventions are effective in large populations.[1] The campaign to persuade Americans to lower their blood cholesterol levels draws on not just one, but many randomized controlled trials. By comparison with screening for cervical cancer, where a trial has never been done, and screening for prostate cancer, where there is only one small trial of treatment, the research on high blood cholesterol is rich in well-designed trials.

The Lipid Research Clinics Coronary Primary Prevention Trial, a seven-year trial that enrolled 3,806 high-cholesterol men between the ages of 35 and 59, was hailed as the first to show definitively that *lowering* blood cholesterol could lower the rate of heart disease.[2] The researchers reported that giving a drug, cholestyramine, to half the men cut their rate of heart attacks (fatal and nonfatal combined) by 19 percent compared with the men who did not receive the drug. Years of population studies, clinical research, and experiments in animals had identified cholesterol as a factor in heart disease. Here was strong evidence, in humans, to support taking action.

The National Institutes of Health (NIH) convened a conference of experts the same year to draw up recommendations about what should be done. In line with the experts' advice, NIH created the National Cholesterol Education Program (NCEP) in 1985 to serve as a permanent advisory body and to develop detailed guidelines for the medical profession and the public. NCEP's Adult Treatment Panel published its recommendations for screening and treatment in January 1988.[3]

The panel recommended that all adults twenty or older have their blood cholesterol levels checked at least every five years. Levels between 200 and 239 milligrams per deciliter (mg/dl) were termed "borderline high," while levels 240 mg/dl or above were "high" cholesterol. People with high cholesterol, and those with borderline high cholesterol who already had heart disease—or two or more other risk factors for heart disease—would undergo a second blood test to determine their level of low-density-lipoprotein (LDL) cholesterol (a component of total blood cholesterol, popularly known as "bad" cholesterol). LDL cholesterol is usually, but not always, high when total cholesterol is high. Additional risk factors for heart disease include being male, smoking, high blood pressure, diabetes, being 30 percent or more overweight, a family history of premature heart disease, a personal history of stroke or peripheral vascular disease, and a low level of high-density-lipoprotein (HDL) cholesterol (another component of total blood cholesterol, known as "good" cholesterol).

The goal for treatment was to reduce LDL cholesterol. A low-fat diet (Step I) was recommended as the first step in treatment, with an even lower-fat diet (Step II) if that was not successful. If LDL cholesterol was high enough and six months to a year of diet did not work, physicians were advised to consider cholesterol-lowering drugs in addition to diet. The diet, and probably the drugs, would have to be maintained for a lifetime. The panel recommended that, once the best pattern of treatment was established, the physician should see patients on diet twice a year and those on diet and drugs every four months.

The potential size of the effort was huge. There are more than 175 million people twenty or older in the United States.[4] More than half have cholesterol levels above 200 mg/dl.[5] By design, the cutoff point for high cholesterol, 240 mg/dl, was chosen to include one-quarter of the adult population, and thus 25 percent of those screened would be diagnosed as high cholesterol and at least another 25 percent would be labeled borderline high. It has been estimated that, after LDL cholesterol levels and risk factors are determined, 36 percent of the adult population would require diet and/or drugs.[6]

Cholesterol had already become a household word thanks to the efforts of the American Heart Association. With publication of the NCEP guidelines, most Americans quickly learned that their blood cholesterol was supposed to be less than 200 mg/dl and that they should see a doctor to have it checked. Surveys showed that, in 1983, 35 percent of adults had had their cholesterol tested; by 1990 that number had risen to 65 percent.[7] Food manufacturers catered to the new concern, adding prominent labels to low cholesterol items (and thereby helping to confuse the public, which did not always realize that the dietary target was all fats, particularly saturated fats and cholesterol, not just cholesterol[8]).

"The Cholesterol Myth"

In 1989 the steady flow of articles about the role of cholesterol in heart disease and the desirability of a low-fat diet was interrupted by a cover story in the September issue of the *Atlantic* titled "The Cholesterol Myth."[9] The blurb on the cover succinctly summarized the main points: "Lowering your cholesterol is next to impossible with diet, and often dangerous with drugs—and it won't make you live any longer." The accompanying picture showed a balding man, mouth taped, restraining himself with obvious effort from tucking into steak, french fries, ice cream, and other high-fat foods. Inside, author Thomas Moore chronicled the arguments that had, until then, taken place in the medical journals out of public view.[10]

The article and the controversy were picked up by the major newspapers. The *New York Times* interviewed experts on both sides.[11] One who had attended the National Institutes of Health Conference in 1984 and had, with others, pointed out the lack of evidence that reducing cholesterol helped anyone live longer reported, "We were as welcome as ants at a picnic." On its editorial page, the *Times* noted that the patients in the trials who received cholesterol-lowering drugs "suffered less heart disease than an untreated group but, oddly enough, didn't live any longer."[12] The term "oddly enough" sounded a dismissive note that appeared in other stories, and which reflected the views of many of the experts who supported the National Cholesterol Education Program.

Time, Reader's Digest, and *Consumer Reports* all carried stories prompted by the article in the *Atlantic*.[13] They gave more attention to Moore's arguments that diet was not an effective way to lower cholesterol, and that the possible risks of taking cholesterol-lowering drugs for a lifetime were not known, than to the statement that lowering cholesterol would not help anyone live longer. When *Time* and *Consumer Reports* did mention that finding, they labeled it "puzzling," and *Time* reported that it did "not overly impress most researchers." The *Reader's Digest* article ended with a summary of the medical research that included the watered-down statement that "the evidence that they [cholesterol-lowering drugs and diets] extend life is not conclusive.'' And then the story faded from the front page and from the minds of most Americans.

The Accumulating Evidence

Reports from the clinical trials and the National Cholesterol Education Program typically state that reducing blood cholesterol has been shown to reduce the rate of heart attacks and death from heart disease and stop there, leaving the impression that people live longer as a result. The full truth, that lowering cholesterol has been found to reduce the rate of heart disease, but not to extend life, is another one of those statements that, after all the years of publicity to the contrary, sounds hopelessly nonsensical. How could it possibly reduce deaths from heart disease without also extending life? The answer: by causing more deaths from other diseases, enough to match the reduction in heart disease deaths. Cholesterol reduction is a double-edged sword, with bad effects as well as good ones.

When it appeared in the early trials, the finding was so unexpected that it was passed off as probably nothing more than a chance occurrence, one of those quirky things that happens once in a while. But the research on cholesterol reduction is rich in randomized controlled trials, and as the results have continued to come in, and to be compared across studies, the same finding has appeared over and over again: Reducing blood cholesterol is associated with an increase in deaths from causes other than heart disease that cancels the decline in heart disease deaths. Again and again, the same trials that have shown that lowering cholesterol reduces deaths from heart disease have also shown that lowering cholesterol does not make people live longer.

In 1990, almost exactly a year after Moore's article in the

Atlantic, an analysis of six trials of cholesterol reduction appeared in the *British Medical Journal.*[14] All six trials were randomized and controlled. All studied healthy populations and are thus relevant to the issue of whether cholesterol reduction is useful for the general population. Since most of the trial participants were men, only the results for men were used in the analysis. The trials tested cholesterol reduction by means of diet or drugs. Trials that combined cholesterol reduction with other interventions, such as programs to help men stop smoking, were omitted because it is not possible to tell which intervention produced which changes.[15]

All six trials consistently failed to show that reducing cholesterol extended life. The total number of deaths in the treated groups (the groups on diet or drugs) was actually larger than the number in the control groups, although the excess was small enough that it might have been due to chance. Only one of the trials had, by itself, been able to show a reduction in deaths from heart disease that passed conventional statistical tests. Others that individually reported statistically significant reductions were able to do so because they added nonfatal heart attacks to deaths from heart disease and tested the total, rather than the component parts. The analysis of all six trials showed that the decline in deaths from heart disease was almost, but not quite, large enough to satisfy the usual statistical tests.

The authors then examined deaths from causes other than heart disease to try to determine which ones had increased in the treated groups. Some evidence has suggested that lowering cholesterol might lead to more deaths from cancer, but the results showed this to be the problem in only one of the six trials—the World Health Organization trial in which Clofibrate, a drug that has been associated with higher rates of cancer, was used. Instead, and consistently and strongly across all six trials, the treated groups suffered more deaths from accidents, suicide, and homicide. The rate of death from these causes was almost twice as high in the treated as in the control groups, and cancelled the reduction in heart disease deaths. The authors noted that "compared with control subjects, treated groups had 28 fewer deaths per 100,000 from coronary heart disease and 29 excess deaths from suicides, homicides, and accidents."

Other analyses of large numbers of trials have also found more deaths from causes other than heart disease in the groups that lowered their blood cholesterol levels, but have not been able to identify specific causes of death as the problem.[16] But because these studies combined trials of healthy people with trials of people who had suffered heart attacks, they are not as pertinent to the issue of screening for healthy people. At the same time, they muddy the findings for survivors of heart attacks, for which cholesterol reduction has been shown to be more clearly beneficial.

Medical experts do not know what physiological processes might explain the increase in deaths from causes other than heart disease. Since cholesterol is essential to many bodily functions, explanations may well exist, but the issue is largely unexplored.[17] As one recent editorial notes, however, the lack of a biological explanation is not reason enough to ignore the result. "Statistically significant results in randomized trials strongly suggest causality," and the suggestion is as valid when cholesterol appears to cause an increase in deaths from other causes as when it appears to cause a decrease in deaths from heart disease.[18]

The authors of the NCEP guidelines knew that trials in healthy populations had not shown that people lived longer. To support their belief that reducing blood cholesterol would lead to longer life, they referred instead to a trial that enrolled survivors of heart attacks, the Coronary Drug Project.[19] Many trials have been done on heart-attack patients, more than on healthy people, because the rate of subsequent heart attacks among men who have suffered one is so high that the chance of making a difference over a short period of time is much greater. The Coronary Drug Project, the largest of these trials, had tested five different drugs; three were discontinued early because death rates were higher in the groups receiving them than in the control group.[20] When the trial ended after six years, one of the two remaining drugs—niacin (a B vitamin)—had shown modest benefit in reducing the rate of repeat heart attacks. Fifteen years after the beginning of the trial, and nine years after its end, the men who had taken niacin had benefited from 11 percent fewer deaths from all causes than the men in the control group. Thus it was concluded that the intervention that had ended nine years earlier had something to do with the reduction.

In 1990 an analysis of eight trials in heart-attack patients was published that, like the one of trials in healthy people, used special statistical techniques for generalizing across different trials.[21] Taken together, the trials showed definitively that deaths from heart attack had been reduced in the treated groups, as had nonfatal heart attacks. The difference in deaths from all causes was "favorable"—that is, there were fewer deaths in the groups on diet or drugs than in the control groups—but not large enough to dismiss the possibility that it might have occurred by chance. Total deaths fell less than heart disease deaths because, as in the studies of healthy populations, the treated groups suffered more deaths from other causes. Since, however, heart disease is far and away the dominant cause of death for people who have survived one heart attack, the increase was not enough to offset entirely the drop in heart disease deaths.

In the absence of evidence that reducing blood cholesterol lengthens the lives of people who do not already have heart disease, supporters and critics of the cholesterol campaign have engaged in a variety of arguments.[22]

Supporters point to evidence from population studies showing that, at least in middle-aged men, naturally low cholesterol levels are associated with lower total mortality. Critics respond that this does not prove that reducing the cholesterol of those whose levels are naturally high will produce the same results, and the clinical trials give reason to suspect it will not.

Supporters argue that the results for heart-attack patients indicate the potential benefits for other people. Critics respond that more than 80 percent of deaths in this group are from heart disease, so that adverse effects that operate through other diseases have much less chance to cancel heart-disease gains than in other groups in the population.

Supporters argue that the trials did not last long enough to demonstrate the benefits of cholesterol reduction. Critics respond that this assumes that only the benefits, not the adverse effects, would grow larger with time. The adverse effects might also grow larger, continuing to cancel the benefits.

Supporters argue that cholesterol reduction is unlikely to be the reason for the failure to find fewer total deaths because no specific causes appear to be the problem in every trial. Critics respond that recent studies call this into question as they begin to identify more specific causes—such as accidents, suicide, and homicide—across trials.

Supporters argue that the trials were not large enough
to show a benefit in terms of deaths from all causes.
Critics respond that, since there are more deaths from
all causes than from heart disease in every trial, trials
large enough to show a difference in heart disease
deaths are large enough to show one in deaths from
all causes. In advancing this argument, supporters are
thus granting the existence of at least some adverse
effects from cholesterol reduction, which offset the
benefits, thus making any difference in deaths from all
causes smaller and harder to detect.

Supporters argue that, even if it does not make people
live longer, cholesterol reduction will make the years
lived healthier since it has been proven to reduce
heart attacks. Critics respond that this claim ignores
not only the significant side effects of drugs but also
the ill health that may accompany the larger number
of deaths from other causes. None of the trials has
attempted to examine this question by comparing the
overall health of men receiving diet and drugs with
that of men in the control group.

Supporters argue that, with heart disease the number
one cause of death in the United States—500,000
deaths every year—it is essential to do something
even if the evidence is imperfect. Critics respond that
anything recommended for the entire adult population
has the potential to do a great deal of harm as well as
a great deal of good. Premature action could produce
more harm than good.

In spite of all the randomized controlled trials, the cholesterol campaign is based not on incontrovertible scientific evi-

dence that cholesterol reduction is beneficial, but on educated guesses, on pieces of evidence that suggest it might be. A different set of guesses, equally educated, leads to the conclusion that cholesterol reduction could be beneficial for people who have had heart attacks, but not for other people, and that it might even be harmful for some.

Women, Children, and the Elderly

Most of the participants in the trials of healthy people were middle-aged men with very high levels of blood cholesterol. Population studies show that the link between cholesterol and heart disease is strongest for this group and that the incidence of heart disease rises rapidly as cholesterol levels rise.[23] Thus the efficacy of reducing cholesterol should be most easily demonstrated in middle-aged men with high levels. Critics have questioned using the results of these trials to make policies for the elderly, women, children, and young men, or, for that matter, middle-aged men with less than the highest cholesterol levels. Even if cholesterol reduction is beneficial for middle-aged men with very high levels, the benefit is likely to be less, or nonexistent, in these groups, exactly because cholesterol plays a smaller role.

Nonetheless the recommendations of the National Cholesterol Education Program, and of other groups, include the old, the young, and women. The NCEP noted that cholesterol was a less important risk factor in these groups. Rather than exempting them from the guidelines, however, the NCEP allowed that "there is room for modifications based on the judgment of the physician and the preferences of the patient when dealing with individual patients, particularly young adults, the elderly, and women."[24]

Because blood cholesterol levels rise with age, but the NCEP cutoff points for borderline high and high cholesterol do not, a large number of elderly people are candidates for treatment. The advisability of screening the elderly was reviewed by the Office of Technology Assessment (OTA) when Congress considered paying for cholesterol screening under Medicare.[25] OTA found that, in men over 65, high blood cholesterol is no longer associated with more deaths from heart disease. In elderly women, although high cholesterol is linked with more deaths from heart disease, it does not shorten their lives. Indeed, some research indicates that elderly people with high blood cholesterol may live longer than those with lower cholesterol.

The report noted that no trials have been conducted of cholesterol reduction in the elderly. Because many of the elderly have chronic conditions (often more than one) and take several prescription drugs, and because their responses to drugs differ from those of younger people, they are likely to suffer more side effects from cholesterol-lowering drugs. Unless cholesterol reduction confers substantial benefit to offset the side effects, it might thus do them real harm. Nor is diet a riskless alternative. A past president of the American Heart Association has expressed dismay that, because they are fearful of eating anything that might raise their cholesterol levels, some elderly people end up malnourished.[26] Mindful of this possibility, the NCEP recommended against intensive dietary therapy (the Step II diet) in "most" elderly patients.[27]

Screening and treatment of children is especially controversial. No trials have been conducted in children. The NCEP, along with the American Academy of Pediatrics, is relatively conservative in recommending only that children over the age of two in families with a history of premature heart disease, or who have one parent with high blood cholesterol, be screened.[28] By this guideline, about one in four children would be screened. The goal is to treat those who have elevated LDL-cholesterol levels with diet and possibly drugs. Other groups, however, have called for screening all children with the aim of treating elevated levels.[29] So far children under the age of two have been exempted from the debate since it is generally agreed that nature seems to have intended them to have a high-fat diet; 50 percent of the calories in human breast milk come from fat.[30]

Screening children raises important questions about the strength of the link between childhood and adult cholesterol levels, the very long-term effects of treatment, and the effects of low-fat diets and cholesterol-reducing drugs during childhood. Cholesterol levels in childhood are only loosely related to adult levels, and cholesterol levels in adulthood are imperfectly related to heart disease; many adults with elevated levels never get heart disease. One study tracked 2,367 children between the ages of eight and eighteen until they reached adulthood to determine which of those with elevated cholesterol levels in childhood had levels as adults high enough to warrant treatment according to the NCEP recommendations.[31] Of the one-quarter with the highest childhood levels, only 25 percent of the girls and 44 percent of the boys still had elevated levels in adulthood. Had they been treated as children, 75 percent of the girls and 56 percent of the boys would have been treated unnecessarily. Even among the top 10 percent of the children, large numbers no longer had elevated levels by the time they reached adulthood: 57 percent of the girls and 30 percent of the boys would have been treated unnecessarily.

Recommendations for childhood screening implicitly assume that treatment is more effective the earlier it begins. This is a general premise behind all prevention—later may be too late because the condition cannot be reversed.[32] There is, however, no evidence for the effectiveness of treating children. The treatment trials in adults, both healthy adults and those with heart disease, suggest that the condition can be reversed—blood cholesterol can be reduced in adulthood, and with it the risk of heart disease. Thus current evidence suggests that it may be just as effective to wait. Indeed, since better treatments are likely to be developed in the future, it may be preferable to wait.[33]

Not only are the potential benefits less for children, the risks of treatment are likely to be greater. Partly, this is because treatment started in childhood is expected to be lifelong. Thus children will be exposed to any adverse effects for fifty or sixty years or more. The Step II diet recommended by the NCEP is so restrictive that careful planning with the help of a dietitian is required to make sure the child gets enough vitamins, minerals, and calories.[34] For children over ten years of age, drug therapy is supposed to be considered when diet does not reduce cholesterol levels sufficiently. The clinical trials have shown that both diet and drugs lead to more deaths from causes other than heart disease. In middle-aged adults the reduction in heart disease deaths offsets the deaths from other causes, leaving life expectancy unchanged. Children and young adults rarely suffer heart disease—their major causes of death are accidents, suicide, and homicide. If the adverse effects of cholesterol reduction are concentrated on exactly these causes, the result in this age group could be "a major tragedy"[35] since there would be no offsetting benefit.

Accuracy of the Test

The extent to which any benefits of cholesterol reduction are realized in practice depends in part on how accurately the blood test identifies individuals' true levels. Under the best of circumstances, blood cholesterol is not a perfect predictor of heart disease. Many people with elevated levels, even those with very high levels, do not develop heart disease and will not benefit from treatment. The potential benefit is further reduced when inaccurate tests mean people are classified as having elevated cholesterol when they do not, or as having desirable cholesterol levels when their true levels are elevated.

Some inaccuracy is unavoidable because individuals' blood cholesterol levels vary substantially from day to day, and month to month.[36] The same individual can easily have a level of 187 mg/dl at one test and 220 at the next.[37] Moreover, cholesterol levels appear to follow a seasonal pattern. In the Lipid Research Clinics trial, the average reading was 7 mg/dl higher in December than in June, suggesting that people whose levels are measured during the winter are at greater risk of being diagnosed as having high cholesterol. To reduce the effect of this variability, the NCEP recommends that a diagnosis be based on the average of at least two tests, taken one to eight weeks apart, with a third test if the first two differ by more than 30 mg/dl.[38]

The risk of misclassification is increased by the poor quality of work done by many laboratories. The labs involved in clinical trials use a method for measuring blood cholesterol—the modified Abel-Kendall method—which is considered the most accurate, and also the most difficult, and they pay close attention to maintaining accuracy.[39] Most labs use less accurate methods and are less careful about maintaining standards. In 1985 the American College of Pathologists sent blood samples with a known cholesterol value of 262.6 mg/dl to five thousand laboratories.[40] The laboratories reported back results ranging from 101 to 524. Even after the 107 most extreme values were eliminated, the range was 187 to 379. Surveys in 1986 and 1987 produced similar results.

Final diagnosis and treatment decisions are based on the level of LDL cholesterol. LDL cholesterol is not measured directly but is calculated from the results for total blood cholesterol, HDL cholesterol, and triglycerides. Most authorities agree that HDL-cholesterol determinations are less accurate than those of total cholesterol, and thus LDL tests are less accurate.[41] The consequence of all these inaccuracies is that, in the real world, patients will be misclassified more often than they are in clinical trials, and thus any possible benefit from cholesterol reduction will be less.

The NCEP recommends that physicians use additional tests of total blood cholesterol to monitor the effect of diet and drugs once treatment begins. Depending on the test results, the physician decides whether diet alone is successful, or, if drugs are necessary, which ones work best. But an article on how to interpret test results in light of individual and laboratory variation concludes that the results are too unreliable to guide treatment.[42] Someone who is responding well can nonetheless easily produce readings showing no change or even a small increase in cholesterol. The authors suggest that the physician and patient simply have to proceed on the assumption that, if treatment has been shown to work for patients in general, it is working for this patient.

Potential Benefits

Suppose it is eventually shown that cholesterol reduction is good for everyone, making it possible to live longer, healthier lives. What would the gain in life expectancy look like? To answer this question, Taylor and colleagues used the evidence from a population study, the Framingham Heart Study, which shows that people with naturally low blood cholesterol levels live longer than those with higher levels.[43] Based on these data, they estimated how much longer people with high cholesterol might expect to live if they lowered their cholesterol levels by 3 percent, 6.7 percent, and 20 percent.[44]

The gains in life expectancy were uniformly small for people with no risk factors other than high cholesterol, ranging from three days to three months, depending on age, sex, and initial cholesterol levels. The numbers are averages for all people with the same characteristics. They could be the result of small gains for everyone, larger gains for a few while most gain nothing, or even large gains for some while others' lives are shortened. But because the averages are low, it is clear that few people could hope for large gains in life expectancy.

For people with risk factors in addition to high blood cholesterol—high blood pressure, smoking, and low HDL cholesterol—the potential gains are larger, at least for fairly substantial reductions in cholesterol (Table 3). If the average reduction in cholesterol were 20 percent, the gain in life expectancy for all groups except sixty-year-old men could be as much as a year or even two. For reductions of only 3 percent, the potential gains are only a few months. Taylor and colleagues present additional estimates to show that the gains in life expectancy from quitting smoking or reducing blood pressure are considerably larger for most of these groups.

The estimates represent possible, not actual, gains since clinical trials have not shown that cholesterol reduction lengthens life. They can be thought of as the most that could be achieved if individuals adopted a low-fat diet and the diet had no adverse effects. The potential gains would be less if cholesterol levels were reduced through screening and treatment along the lines of the NCEP recommendations—because people would be misclassified by the test more often in everyday medical practice than were subjects in the Framing-

Table 3   Months Added to Life Expectancy of High-Risk People by Reduction of Blood Cholesterol

	If Diet Reduces Blood Cholesterol by		
	3%	6.7%	20%
For women age			
20	2	4	12
40	4	9	24
60	5	11	29
For men age			
20	2	4	11
40	3	7	18
60	1	2	5

NOTE: High-risk people are defined as smokers with blood pressure and total blood cholesterol levels equal to or higher than those of 90 percent of people of their age and sex (the 90th percentile), and HDL cholesterol lower than that of all but 10 percent of people of their age and sex (the 10th percentile). The estimates assume that it takes three years for cholesterol reduction to reduce the individual's risk of heart disease to the risk associated with the new, lower cholesterol level.

SOURCE: William C. Taylor, Theodore M. Pass, Donald S. Shepard, and Anthony L. Komaroff, "Cholesterol Reduction and Life Expectancy: A Model Incorporating Multiple Risk Factors," *Annals of Internal Medicine* 106 (April 1987): Table 2.

ham Study and because of the side effects of cholesterol-lowering drugs.

Many people who take drugs experience daily side effects that make the years of life on treatment, as well as the months gained, less pleasant. The bile acid sequestrants (Cholestyramine and Colestipol) cause gastrointestinal problems, niacin causes flushing and itching of the skin, and the fibric acids (Clofibrate and Gemfibrozil) increase the risk of gallstones.[45] Lovastatin is currently thought to have few side effects, but its safety over a period of several years is not known. One study has calculated that small side effects over many years can substantially reduce the potential benefit from cholesterol reduction.[46]

Costs and Potential Cost-Effectiveness

Garber and Wagner have estimated the costs of achieving full compliance with the NCEP guidelines for all adults without heart disease in the United States.[47] As prescribed by the guidelines, all adults are assumed to be screened and those with elevated cholesterol receive treatment with diet and, if necessary, with drugs as well, to reduce their LDL cholesterol to the recommended levels. The effectiveness of diet in lowering cholesterol is crucial to the expense of treatment since, when diet is more effective, fewer people require drugs. Two alternative assumptions were used for the estimates—that diet reduces LDL cholesterol by 5 percent and by 10 percent.[48]

The costs include the costs of screening, subsequent physician visits, cholesterol-lowering drugs, and extra tests recommended for people on drugs, and are made separately for different drugs. The estimates are on the low side because they assume that the visit at which the first test takes place occurs for some other reason, and so exclude its cost, and because they omit the costs of dietary counseling, although NCEP recommends counseling. They also exclude the costs of treating high cholesterol in people who already have heart disease.

The total costs are large, ranging from $8 billion to $66 billion, depending on the effectiveness of diet and the specific medication used (Table 4). For niacin, the least expensive

Table 4   Annual Costs of the NCEP Recommendations
(in billions of 1991 dollars)

If the Drug is	If LDL Reduction from Diet is	
	5 Percent	10 Percent
Niacin	$ 11.6	$ 8.4
Lovastatin, 20 mg daily	27.3	19.5
Lovastatin, 80 mg daily	66.6	47.2

NOTE: Costs are estimated for the projected number of adults age 20 or older in 1995 without heart disease at the time of initial screening.

SOURCE: Alan M. Garber and Judith L. Wagner, "Practice Guidelines and Cholesterol Policy," *Health Affairs* 10 (Summer 1991): exhibit 2.

drug, costs are $11.6 billion when diet reduces cholesterol by 5 percent, and $8.4 billion when it is more successful. But niacin's unpleasant side effects discourage many people from taking the prescribed doses. Lovastatin, a drug so new that it was not available for use in the major clinical trials, is currently the most popular of the cholesterol-lowering drugs. Thus the estimates for Lovastatin are probably a more accurate indication of the costs of the NCEP guidelines. When Lovastatin is the drug of choice, costs range from $19 billion at doses of 20 milligrams daily to $66 billion when the daily dose is 80 milligrams; larger doses produce larger reductions in cholesterol.

If reducing cholesterol could produce the gains in life estimated by Taylor and colleagues, how would the costs and the gains compare? In another study, Taylor and colleagues calculated the cost of saving a year of life through a program of intensive diet therapy, along the lines of the program used in the Multiple Risk Factor Intervention Trial (MRFIT).[49] The cost of an additional year of life is high for men who have elevated cholesterol but no other risk factors for heart disease (Fig. 3). For example, diet therapy costs more than $500,000 per year of life for low-risk twenty-year-old men with an initial cholesterol of 240 mg/dl. For high-risk men, those with several other risk factors, costs are much lower. They range from a high of $99,000 per year saved for young men with an initial cholesterol level of 240 mg/dl to a low of $11,000 per year for middle-aged men with an initial cholesterol of 300 mg/dl.

Goldman and colleagues compared the use of Lovastatin to treat healthy people with its use for people who had already suffered a heart attack.[50] Like Taylor and colleagues, they found that, for healthy people, the cost of saving a year of life is much higher for those with high blood cholesterol as their only risk factor than for those with several risk factors, even when cholesterol is very high—300 mg/dl (Fig. 4). Lovastatin was even less cost-effective for people with cholesterol levels of 250 to 299 mg/dl. Their analysis also shows that it is potentially much more cost-effective to treat people who have had heart attacks. For some in this category, such as men ages thirty-five to forty-four, drug treatment might save money as well as lives. For all heart-attack survivors, the cost per year of life saved is relatively low.

To make their calculations, both Taylor and Goldman assumed the best, that cholesterol reduction extends lives in direct proportion to the number of heart-disease deaths prevented, and that it has no adverse effects. They also underestimated costs by omitting the costs of initial screening to identify people in need of treatment, and, in the Goldman study, by omitting the costs of dietary therapy, which is recommended in conjunction with drugs. Their results suggest that, even when given its best shot, cholesterol reduction is a very expensive way to save lives for many people. It has the potential to be worthwhile in patients who have suffered heart

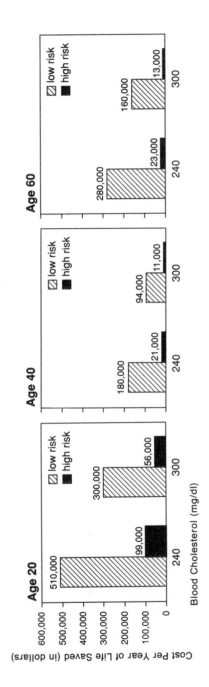

Figure 3. Cost per Year of Life Saved by Diet Notes: Diet is assumed to reduce initial blood cholesterol levels by 6.7%, the average reduction in the MRFIT trial. Costs (in 1986 dollars) and health gains are discounted at 5% per year. Discounting is the process by which costs paid and benefits received in the near term are given more weight than those that occur in the distant future; the higher the discount rate, the less weight given future costs and benefits. A low-risk man is a nonsmoker with systolic blood pressure lower than all but 10% and HDL cholesterol equal to or higher than 90% of men of the same age. A high-risk man is a smoker with systolic blood pressure equal to or higher than 90% and HDL cholesterol lower than all but 10% of men of the same age. *Source:* William C. Taylor, Theodore M. Pass, Donald S. Shepard, and Anthony L. Komaroff, "Cost Effectiveness of Cholesterol Reduction for the Primary Prevention of Coronary Heart Disease in Men," in Richard B. Goldbloom and Robert S. Lawrence, eds., *Preventing Disease: Beyond the Rhetoric* (New York: Springer-Verlag, 1990), Table 44.3.

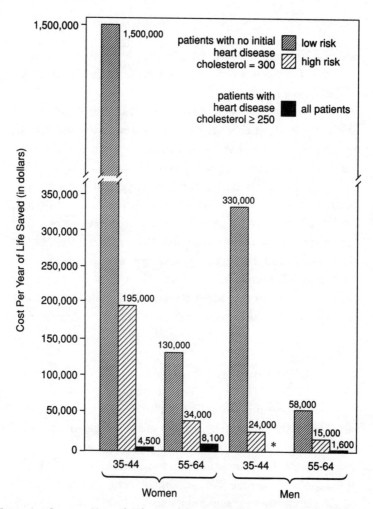

Figure 4. Cost per Year of Life Saved by Lovastatin Notes: Dose is 20 mg of Lovastatin daily. Costs (in 1989 dollars) include physician visits and tests required to monitor people taking Lovastatin. Costs and health gains are discounted at 5% per year (see notes to fig. 3 for a definition of discounting). A low-risk person is a non-smoker with diastolic blood pressure below 95 mm Hg and not more than 10% overweight. A high-risk person is a smoker with a diastolic pressure of 105 mm Hg or higher and 30% or more overweight. * = Lovastatin estimated to save lives and money. *Source:* Lee Goldman, Milton C. Weinstein, Paula A. Goldman, and Lawrence W. Williams, "Cost-Effectiveness of HMG-CoA Reductase Inhibition for Primary and Secondary Prevention of Coronary Heart Disease," *Journal of the American Medical Association* 265 (March 6, 1991), Tables 1–4.

attacks, and in high-risk patients, but is probably not cost-effective for many of the low-risk patients included in the NCEP guidelines.

The Toronto Working Group on Cholesterol Policy has stated the costs of cholesterol reduction in a way that speaks directly to patients.[51] Working from the evidence of the clinical trials, and ignoring the increase in deaths from other causes, they estimated the number of patient-years of drug treatment necessary to prevent one death from heart disease. About 1,100 years of treatment were required in the Lipid Research Clinics trial, more than 1,900 years of treatment in the Helsinki trial. For elderly people, young men, women, and people with lower cholesterol levels than those of the men in the trials, it would take many thousands of years of treatment to prevent one death from heart disease.

A Population Strategy?

Clinical policymakers on all sides of the cholesterol issue agree that a campaign to persuade the general population to reduce the fat content of its diet is a good idea.[52] A major reason for promoting this population approach is the concern that recommendations aimed at high-risk people, like NCEP's guidelines for screening and treatment, will not benefit the majority of those who ultimately die from heart disease because they are not sufficiently high-risk. Support for a population strategy rests as well on the assumptions that a change in diet is riskless, inexpensive, and avoids the problems created when some people can eat foods that are forbidden to others.

In 1991 an NCEP panel published a report recommending that all Americans over the age of two restrict their fat intake to 30 percent of calories or less.[53] The authors noted that more deaths from heart disease occur in people with cholesterol levels below 240 mg/dl than in people with higher levels. They reviewed the evidence showing that the death rate from heart disease is lower for people with naturally low levels of blood cholesterol and that the relationship is continuously graded; that is, there is no point at which cholesterol level no longer seems to matter—the lower the level, the lower the death rate from heart disease. Continuous grading is one sign that a relationship is truly one of cause and effect. In addition, data from the Framingham study and MRFIT show fewer deaths from all causes among people with lower cholesterol levels. People with levels in the neighborhood of 180 mg/dl lived the longest.

That people with naturally low cholesterol levels live longer does not prove that reducing the cholesterol of people with naturally elevated levels will help them live longer. That is why clinical trials were necessary to test the effect of cholesterol reduction. NCEP's population panel was aware that "overall mortality has tended to remain unchanged" in the trials of both diet and drugs. It also recognized that studies had suggested that the risk of death increases at levels of blood cholesterol below 180 mg/dl. The panel concluded, however, that the risks were "either nonexistent or very small." On the strength of the population relationships between heart disease and cholesterol, and the trial evidence that lowering cholesterol lowers the rates of heart disease, the panel recommended a low-fat diet for everyone.

But evidence that low levels of cholesterol are associated with higher death rates has continued to accumulate. Data on 361,662 men screened for MRFIT show that deaths decline until cholesterol is about 180 mg/dl, then rise again at lower cholesterol levels.[54] Here again, the relationship observed in populations does not prove that reducing people's cholesterol levels into this range would cause them to suffer higher death rates. Still, it raises the possibility that a population strategy could harm people with already low levels of cholesterol. Since screening is not required, these people would not be identified and warned to avoid changing their diet.

An extensive review of the risks associated with low cholesterol was published in 1992, the product of a National Institutes of Health conference. The conference participants analyzed the evidence from nineteen different studies with a combined enrollment of 523,737 men and 124,814 women.[55] Men and women were analyzed separately and comparisons were made for four broad groupings of blood cholesterol levels: less than 160 mg/dl; 160 to 199 mg/dl; 200 to 239 mg/dl; and 240 or more mg/dl.

The results, based on studies conducted in the United States, Europe, Israel, and Japan, were impressive in their consistency. For men, the relationship between blood cholesterol and deaths from all causes was U-shaped; in study after study, there were more deaths in the lowest group, as well as the highest group, compared with the two middle groups. More important, the rise in deaths was just as large for the lowest group as the highest. Heart disease was, of course, the reason for the high death rate in men with cholesterol levels 240 or higher. For men with levels under 160, the causes of the extra deaths were identified as cancers other than colon cancer, respiratory disease, digestive disease, and trauma (accidents, suicide, and homicide).

The conference participants took steps to determine whether the relationships were cause and effect or mere chance associations. Deaths during the first five years after each study began were omitted from the analyses because some diseases may cause, rather than be caused by, low cho-

lesterol. Omitting these early deaths was expected to elimi-
nate most cases in which unsuspected disease might have
been the reason for a low cholesterol reading at the start of the
study. The participants also examined whether the relationship between cholesterol and deaths from each cause was
continuously graded. Deaths from cancers other than colon
cancer, respiratory disease, and digestive disease showed a
continuously graded risk, but those from trauma did not—
while they were highest in the low-cholesterol group, there
was little difference among the three higher groups.

The conference could not examine whether deaths from
these causes were also more numerous at cholesterol levels
somewhat above 160 mg/dl, a possibility suggested by the
MRFIT data cited earlier. The cutoff point of 160 mg/dl for
the lowest group helped to sharpen the differences between it
and the others, but ruled out the possibility of testing whether
the relationship extended into this higher range.

For women, the results were the same for specific causes of
death. Death rates from cancers other than colon cancer,
respiratory disease, and digestive disease were higher in the
low-cholesterol group and showed a graded relationship with
cholesterol across the four groups. Deaths from trauma were
higher only in the lowest group. Yet the overall result for
women was quite different. Although deaths from all causes
were modestly higher for the low-cholesterol group, there
were no differences among the three higher groups. The
U-shaped pattern found for men did not extend to women.

The population approach is even more a matter of educated guesses than the medical approach, which focuses on
high-risk people. Its appeal lies to a great extent in the sense
that a low-fat diet "can't hurt and might help." But the clinical trial evidence raises doubts about whether it will help—
clinical trials of diet have gotten results no better, indeed not

as good, as those of drugs. And the impressively consistent evidence on the risks of low cholesterol levels suggests that it could do real harm to some people. The current scientific evidence for a population approach is a weak foundation for changing the lives of millions.

The Best Bet

In light of the evidence, the arguments, and the momentum of the National Cholesterol Education Program, what should individuals and policymakers do?

One reader of a draft of this book asked, "The men in my family tend to die of heart attacks in their early fifties. Will lowering my cholesterol help me avoid that fate?" The answer is not clear. The clinical trial evidence suggests that for men who have already had a heart attack, and thus possibly for men who are at very high risk of heart disease for other reasons, reducing cholesterol reduces the death rate from heart disease and may lengthen life. A man with elevated cholesterol and a family history of premature death from heart disease has three risk factors according to the NCEP guidelines,[56] and cholesterol is the only one he can change. He might decide that lowering his cholesterol somewhat is a reasonable bet— at least to the extent that it can be accomplished through diet. Whether cholesterol-lowering drugs are a good idea if diet alone is not sufficient is a more difficult decision, in light of their unpleasant side effects and the scanty information about their long-term safety. But he could reasonably choose to interpret the evidence as showing that reducing cholesterol will not shorten his life and might lengthen it.[57]

Anyone else, however, should probably interpret the data differently. Cholesterol reduction has not been shown to lengthen life and may shorten it—at considerable trouble and cost. For example, a woman with a family history of cancer and a blood cholesterol that is already below 200 mg/dl has good reason to avoid reducing her cholesterol. She could reasonably ignore the general advice to adopt a low-fat diet. The evidence has not shown the diet to be beneficial for women, and lower cholesterol levels are associated with higher death rates from many cancers as well as other causes.

In addition, there seems to be no persuasive reason for parents to put their children through the rigors of cholesterol reduction. It can be difficult to keep children properly nourished with low-fat diets, the adverse effects of drugs over periods as long as the decades that would be required are simply unknown, and blood cholesterol can always be reduced once the child is grown, long before heart disease would appear. The time, energy, and resources required for childhood intervention are unlikely to produce better health and could cause harm.

For policymakers the same evidence suggests a strategic retreat from the NCEP recommendations. Even when the best is assumed about their effectiveness, interventions to reduce blood cholesterol are very expensive for low-risk people and even for some high-risk people without heart disease. The investment may be worthwhile for heart-attack patients and possibly for other high-risk people, but for most others it appears, on the basis of the current evidence, that the recommendations are as likely to be harmful as helpful. At the same time they require billions of dollars in resources that could be put to better use elsewhere.

In an editorial that accompanied the report on the risks of low cholesterol, three physicians prominent in the cholesterol debate came to similar conclusions.[58] They concluded that screening and treatment are unwise for women and children and that cholesterol-lowering drugs should not be used except by survivors of heart attacks or other people at a similarly high risk of death from heart disease. They argued that, coming on top of the results of the clinical trials, the new data on the mortality risks associated with low cholesterol "call into question policies built over the past several decades on evidence that focussed only on CHD [coronary heart disease] as the outcome."

5

Conclusions

Screening for cervical cancer, prostate cancer, and high blood cholesterol encompass more than half a dozen commonly used screening tests—the Papanicolaou smear, the digital rectal exam, the prostate-specific antigen (PSA) test, transrectal ultrasound, and the blood tests for total cholesterol, HDL cholesterol, and triglycerides. The Pap smear is recommended for all of the 90 million adult women in the United States, and although current U.S. guidelines permit less frequent screening, many doctors still recommend annual tests.[1] A digital rectal exam, increasingly combined with the PSA test and ultrasound, is recommended annually for the 40 million men over age forty. All adults are urged to have their blood cholesterol levels checked at least every five years. With almost 180 million adults in the United States, 35 to 40 million tests each year are required to meet this goal, even before adding millions of extra tests for people who are checked more often because they are at higher risk, and for follow-up and monitoring.

The screening enterprise is large and its potential for expansion is staggering. Since not everyone is screened at the recommended intervals, screening for cervical cancer, prostate cancer, and high blood cholesterol have substantial room for growth just by themselves—only about 20 percent of men over age forty report having had a rectal exam in the last year, 75 percent of women have had a Pap smear in the last three years, and two-thirds of adults have had their cholesterol checked at some point. And these three represent a much larger universe of tests. The U.S. Preventive Services Task Force developed recommendations for an additional forty-four groups of screening tests, and new tests are brought into clinical use every year.

The numbers hint at the more complex dimensions of the enterprise: the time, as well as physical and emotional energy, required of patients to undergo first the tests and then the follow-up when a test is positive; the time and skills of physicians; and the costs to private and public health insurance programs. A great many lives are affected for better or worse, and many more will be in the future. A great many resources are used to provide tests and follow-up care, and many more will be required in the future. Policies toward screening play a major role in determining the size and shape of the medical sector and its impact on health.

Many of the current recommendations oversimplify or ignore important consequences of screening. Too often they seem to be founded on the attitude expressed by one physician about screening children for high cholesterol: "It's a simple, inexpensive test. Why not?"[2] The question implies that the test—which could be any test—is quick and easy, without risk, certain to be beneficial, and so inexpensive that cost need not be considered. The cases examined in this book show that this view is seriously misleading. As a result, current screening recommendations are often pseudo-truths that omit complexities and tradeoffs of great importance to the people they are meant to benefit.

Does It Work?

The issue of first importance for any screening test is whether it accomplishes anything. A test may detect the condition accurately, but does anything need to be done about the condition, and, if something needs to be done, are any of the available therapies effective? Are they more effective when applied early? Unless early treatment makes a difference, screening is pointless.

The examples of prostate cancer and high blood cholesterol show that these are not idle questions. Nor can patients and clinicians assume that the evidence of effectiveness is beyond doubt if the test has been recommended by a prestigious group. In the case of prostate cancer, autopsy evidence shows that many men who die of other causes have cancers that never produced symptoms. Partly because of this large pool of silent cancers, it is difficult to tell whether current screening and treatment procedures lead to longer life. The best evidence, though scant, suggests that they do not.

The evidence about high blood cholesterol is voluminous and of high quality. A large number of randomized controlled trials show that reducing blood cholesterol reduces the risk of getting heart disease, and probably the risk of dying from it. But the same trials also show a consistent, if as yet unexplained, increase in deaths from other causes among the people whose cholesterol is reduced. The increase is so large that it cancels the drop in heart disease deaths, with the result that people who reduce their cholesterol live no longer than those who do not.[3]

Even when a test leads to effective treatment, it has undesirable effects that should be weighed in deciding who to screen and how often. No test, no matter how carefully performed, is 100 percent accurate. Most recommendations emphasize the fact that, because of this, cases of disease can be missed, and more frequent screening is often recommended to counteract the problem. But tests also produce errors of the opposite kind—they identify people as having the condition when they do not. When a test is performed more often, the result is fewer missed cases of disease but more falsely positive results, so that reducing one kind of mistake increases the other.

Falsely positive results lead to follow-up tests, and because follow-up tests are also not perfect, sometimes to treatment—a sequence that can drain the patient's time and energy, and be painful and risky, without conferring any benefit. False positives were discussed most fully in the chapter on screening for cervical cancer, where it was calculated that, over her lifetime, a woman's chance of one or more false positive Pap smears was much higher than her chance of developing cervical cancer. The problem applies, however, to all screening tests. False positives for prostate cancer can lead to unnecessary surgery, with its risk of death or impotence. False positives for high blood cholesterol can lead to years of unnecessary drug therapy, with the unpleasant side effects that accompany cholesterol-lowering drugs.

A somewhat different, but related, point applies to risk factors like high blood cholesterol. Although screening can detect the risk factor, it cannot identify among the many who have the risk factor those who will benefit from treatment. Thus many must undergo treatment to produce benefits that will accrue to a few. Calculations for middle-aged men with very high blood cholesterol levels indicate that between 1,100 and 1,900 patient-years of drug treatment are required to prevent one death from heart disease. Many more years of treatment would be required for most other groups in the population. Even if cholesterol reduction were beneficial, this burden of treatment represents a substantial human cost. Further, the distinction between risk factor and disease blurs when precursor conditions are identified by screening and treated to prevent the disease, as they are for cervical cancer, or when the disease, as is the case for prostate cancer, often does not have serious consequences.

These human costs—falsely positive tests and treatment that is not beneficial for the individual—are virtually ignored in the development of screening recommendations in the United States. The focus instead is on trying to ensure that no case of disease is missed, which leads to recommendations for more frequent screening—a practice that leads in turn to larger numbers of false positives and more treatment without benefit. That bias has probably been aided and abetted by a simple failure to calculate how many people will experience false positives or unnecessary treatment. Calculations like those presented in the chapter on cervical cancer would go a long way toward dispelling the belief that the numbers are small and the consequences minor.

These problems are exacerbated by a series of management issues. Studies show that many laboratories in the United States produce test results that are wrong by a wide margin. These inaccuracies cause people to be misclassified more often than necessary—as having the disease when they do not, or as not having it when they do—and thereby reduce the value of screening. Concern about inaccurate tests, especially Pap smears, led to the passage of new federal legislation to regulate laboratories in 1988.[4] The Clinical Laboratory Improvement Amendments, which replace legislation that dates back to 1967, regulate on the basis of the tests performed, not who performs them, and bring many labs under federal regulation for the first time, including some 130,000 laboratories in doctors' offices.[5] For each testing specialty the law requires a lab to belong to an approved proficiency testing program, which will check the lab's performance each year by having its staff evaluate samples whose values are known to the program. It took four years to develop a set of final regulations acceptable to all parties, and many of the law's requirements will be phased in over two years, so any improvements will not appear for several years.

The new legislation is particularly detailed in its requirements for Pap smears, and cytologic tests in general, which involve the examination of tissue specimens. Here it supports the tradition of focusing on missed cases of disease by imposing heavier penalties when a case is missed than when a healthy person is mistakenly classified as diseased. While an overall score of 90 percent is required to pass the proficiency test, "a person will fail the test if he or she interprets as negative or benign even one slide that shows a high-grade lesion or cancer."[6] In addition, quality control procedures specify that, for any patient found to have a high-grade lesion or cancer, the lab must recheck all tests read as normal during the previous five years.[7]

Two other issues equally important for effective screening programs, recordkeeping and follow-up, have received very little attention in the United States. The International Agency for Research on Cancer found, for example, that the most effective programs of screening for cervical cancer were those in which a central organization maintained laboratory standards, kept patient records, and sent reminders to patients to come in for tests and follow-up.[8] In the United States, the onus is usually on the patient to remember when to have a test, to decline when it is suggested too often, and to call for test results and follow through with subsequent appointments. Yet these functions are crucial to the effectiveness of screening since its only value is to identify people who need further care. Unless they are correctly identified, and the care is received in time, screening has no useful result.

Costs and Cost-Effectiveness

The high costs of screening are often ignored, indeed unrecognized, by those who develop recommendations. Screening all adult women for cervical cancer—a Pap smear and the visit at which it takes place, but not the follow-up care—costs $6 billion a year if the test is done every year. The cost of screening all men over age fifty for prostate cancer with the currently popular sequence of tests is about $4 billion; it would be higher if men between forty and fifty were included. Estimates of the cost of screening adults without heart disease for high cholesterol include follow-up drug therapy as well as the screening test, and range from about $10 billion to more than $60 billion, depending on the drug used and the number of people for whom diet alone is successful. The high estimates are probably more realistic because the most expensive of the cholesterol-lowering drugs, Lovastatin, is also currently the most popular.

These figures may overestimate current spending since they assume that everyone who should get the test according to current recommendations does get it. At the same time, for several reasons, they substantially underestimate the costs that would be incurred if everyone complied with the recommendations. All of the estimates are based on prices that are several years out of date. Those for cervical cancer and prostate cancer exclude the costs of follow-up, both of false positives and of those who truly have the condition. The estimates for cholesterol screening do not count the cost of the doctor's visit at which the screening test takes place and assume that diet therapy is costless, although the recommendations of the National Cholesterol Education Program include both dietary counseling and extra visits to the doctor to monitor progress.

The figures demonstrate the fallacy of assuming that because a single test is inexpensive, a screening program will be too. Screening involves repeated tests, many if not most of them for people who will never get the condition the test is intended to detect. It involves follow-up tests to try to separate the true from the false positive results and treatment for many of those with positive tests. The inexpensive test is deceiving—the complete costs of screening are high.

The health gained for the money varies widely.[9] The full costs of screening and follow-up care for cervical cancer run about $13,000 for each year of life saved when the Pap smear is done every three years, compared with no screening. Cutting the time between tests from three to two years costs $263,000 for each additional year of life. Annual tests cost more than $1 million for each additional life-year compared with screening every two years. The reason for the steeply rising cost of a life-year is that screening every two years costs 50 percent more than screening every three years, and annual screening costs three times as much, but the extra tests catch only a few more cases of cervical cancer. Screening every three years reduces the death rate by 91 percent, while annual screening reduces it by 93 percent—a gain of two percentage points. Results like these played a central role in the professional argument of the 1980s over an appropriate recommendation for Pap testing.

Studies of the costs and benefits of cholesterol reduction show that, even under optimistic assumptions about its effectiveness, reducing cholesterol with Lovastatin is an expensive way to improve health. The cost is especially high for people without heart disease or other risk factors for heart disease, ranging from $60,000 for each year of life saved up to $1.5 million, depending on age, sex, and initial cholesterol level. For healthy people with several risk factors, the cost of saving a year of life is usually under $100,000, again depending on age, sex, and cholesterol level. But for survivors of heart attacks, both the clinical trial evidence and cost-effectiveness studies suggest that cholesterol reduction is a good investment. For them, it saves lives at low cost; indeed, in some cases, the cost is likely to be outweighed by savings in later medical care. These estimates, for people with and without heart disease, include only the costs of drug therapy and monitoring; the screening necessary to identify patients in need of drug therapy is omitted. Thus, while they are useful for indicating orders of magnitude, they are, like so many of the other cost estimates, on the low side of the truth. Indeed, it is important to keep in mind that estimates of costs and cost-effectiveness tend to be optimistic. As in the case of cholesterol, analysts make the most favorable assumptions about effectiveness and are more likely to leave out items, or underestimate their cost, than to count too many and price them too high.

The cost-effectiveness studies show that it is possible to overinvest in screening and underinvest at the same time. Many women in the United States get Pap smears annually, sometimes more often, while a quarter have not had one in at least three years. Testing the latter group more regularly would bring substantial gains in health at relatively low cost. Similarly, even under favorable assumptions about its beneficial effects, cholesterol reduction is an expensive way to improve health for people who do not have heart disease. Yet it is probably not used enough for people who have already had heart attacks.[10]

The cost-effectiveness results suggest an explanation for the uneasy feeling shared by many people that the huge increases in medical care expenditures in the last several decades are not buying much more health. It's true—they are not. Screening for cervical cancer is effective, but annual screening is only a little more effective than screening every three years, and much more expensive. Screening for prostate cancer has increased in recent years, particularly following the publication of new studies of the prostate-specific antigen test, yet there is no good evidence that the available therapies are effective. Screening of the general population for high blood cholesterol is an expensive phenomenon of the last ten years, and probably contributes nothing to longer life.

An Example of the Complexities

Cost-effectiveness analyses contribute to a more balanced assessment of screening recommendations, but they do not yet incorporate everything of importance to patients, clinicians, and policymakers, especially some of the human costs of screening and follow-up treatment. A recent article in the *Journal of the American Medical Association* illustrates the importance of some of the omissions—particularly years of treatment. In the study, Swedish men diagnosed as having early prostate cancer were treated during the subsequent ten years only when their cancer spread or began to produce symptoms, in sharp contrast to the aggressive approach preferred in the United States.[11] Figure 5 compares the Swedish and U.S. approaches for the fifty-eight men whose cancers were considered suitable for radical prostatectomy.[12]

Under the U.S. approach, all fifty-eight men undergo surgery at once. One dies of the surgery. Of the remainder,

58 patients are diagnosed with prostate cancer and over the next ten years:

U.S.	patient years of treatment
All patients undergo surgery immediately	465
1 dies of surgery	
20 become impotent	(165)
3 have some degree of incontinence	(25)
Sweden	
No patients are treated initially	
29 show progression and are treated	180
29 do not show progression but	40
6 are treated for local problems	

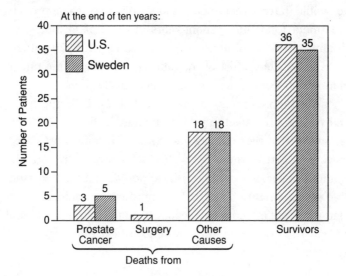

Figure 5.   U.S. and Swedish Approaches to Prostate Cancer

twenty are impotent and three have some degree of incontinence. During the next ten years three die of prostate cancer
and eighteen of other causes, leaving thirty-six survivors.
Under the Swedish approach the men are simply followed. In
half, the cancer progresses and they are treated hormonally,

which can mean either surgery or drugs. In the other half, the disease does not progress, although a few of the men are treated for local problems. Over the ten years, five die of prostate cancer and eighteen of other causes, leaving thirty-five survivors.

At the end of the period the differences amount to a gain of perhaps five years of life in the United States, purchased with an extra two hundred years of treatment. The gain may be less than five years because one man dies immediately from the surgery in the United States, thus losing some life-years that he would have experienced under the Swedish approach. Treatment totals 465 patient-years in the United States, including 165 years of impotence, compared with 220 patient-years in Sweden. Most of the difference is due to the fifteen men who never needed any treatment in Sweden.

As yet there is no good evidence that the U.S. approach, and radical prostatectomy in particular, lengthens life—the life saved is no more than a guesstimate. If radical prostatectomy is effective, there is no "right" answer here, but the example suggests that there is also no easy answer. Reasonable people might choose either approach. If radical prostatectomy is not effective, the example points to the substantial human costs of acting in the absence of evidence.

Patients, Clinicians, and Policymakers

The same issues that arise in screening for cervical cancer, prostate cancer, and high blood cholesterol apply to all screening tests. Their effectiveness can be hard to determine and judgments about it are often based on a patchwork of imperfect evidence, filtered through the beliefs and enthusiasms of the resident experts. Effectiveness aside, all screening tests produce incorrect results some of the time. All require follow-up to try to sort out true cases and treat them, which involves costs spread over so many people and so many separate services that they can appear deceptively small without a careful accounting. All are more beneficial for some people than others.

These general statements, however, are not much use to a patient, clinician, or policymaker faced with making a decision about a particular test. Only careful analysis of the facts will reveal which factors dominate in a particular case. The balance of benefits and costs, both human and resource costs, depends on the nature of the particular disease—the speed of its onset, the nature of its precursor conditions, the seriousness of its consequences, and the characteristics that make people more or less vulnerable to it; on the accuracy of the test in everyday use; on whether treatment is effective, how effective, and when; on the side effects of the tests and treatment; and on the costs at each step and how often they are incurred. The importance of each of these factors differs from one screening test to another. Analyses of the Pap smear or the PSA test cannot show the balance for mammography or blood pressure testing or the myriad of other tests used in modern medicine.

How are patients, clinicians, payers, and policymakers to weigh these factors—years of life saved, falsely positive tests, the burden of treatment, and resource costs—as they face their own decisions? What are they to make of the current recommendations? What might they do to improve them?

Every patient has a clinical practice of one, often more if decisions must also be made about the medical care of children or elderly parents. Patients have a vital interest, literally, in whether tests are valid, whether they lead to effective treatment, and what the risks and benefits of different screening schedules are. Many patients have found themselves facing medical decisions so serious they decided they had to become their own experts. Whether actively or by default, they make the necessary decisions, but they are at a serious disadvantage in getting the information they need and interpreting it in light of their own situations. For most decisions about screening, they must depend in large part on the recommendations of respected medical or governmental groups, with some guidance from their doctors and their own experience. They usually have little way to know whether the recommendations and guidance give them all they would like to know.

Clinicians, although medically trained, are not much better off. They must continually decide which tests to do for which patients, and how to follow them up. Lack of time and lack of training in the methods of inference make it difficult for them to evaluate the evidence correctly and draw their own conclusions. They too must operate primarily on the basis of other experts' recommendations, many of which are absorbed during their initial training and modified, correctly or incorrectly, by their own clinical experience. It is all the easier to accept these recommendations uncritically, or to modify them in the direction of doing even more, when they involve a great deal of work with healthy, compliant, and well-insured patients, permitting clinicians to do well while believing they are also doing good.

For better or worse, both patients and clinicians must continue to depend on policymakers in medical professional groups and government for help. The decisions these groups make about what to recommend and what information to provide about those recommendations largely determine the choices available to patients and clinicians. It is at this level that the major issues having to do with screening must be resolved.

That does not mean that patients or clinicians are limited to acting as passive recipients of whatever recommendations the experts choose. Much of what needs to be changed about the way screening recommendations are developed has to do with the process, the steps that are followed to ensure that everything has been considered that should be, and with open minds. Although the results will differ, the process should be the same from one test to another. By insisting on a high-quality process, and judging the worth of individual recommendations according to whether that process was followed in their development, patients and clinicians can be a powerful force for better screening policies.

Toward Better Screening Policies

Valid recommendations can only come out of a process that ensures that all the evidence is reviewed, important uncertainties are openly discussed, and conclusions are justified by the evidence. It is not enough to get experts together in a room and present them with the results of randomized controlled trials. The momentum created by beliefs, expectations, and years of professional investment in the field can get in the way of evaluating the evidence objectively.

Screening for high blood cholesterol demonstrates the need for a better process. As soon as the Lipid Research Clinics Trial Group published results in 1984 showing that reducing cholesterol reduced the risk of heart disease, experts in the field moved enthusiastically to mount a campaign, led by the National Cholesterol Education Program (NCEP), to persuade Americans to know their cholesterol levels and to lower them by diet, or, if necessary, by drugs. The experts knew that clinical trials had failed to prove that reducing cholesterol would make people live longer. The issue was raised when the NCEP was getting under way, and evidence from a variety of studies supported it as a serious issue, but it was swept aside in the belief that time and future studies would justify the campaign. The costs of the campaign were simply ignored. Time has not brought the expected confirmation, and the costs are large and growing, but the campaign continues.

A committee convened by the Institute of Medicine to consider the development and use of recommendations, or "guidelines" in the committee's terminology, noted the lack of any kind of quality control as a serious drawback of most efforts: "Few guidelines today provide any formal projections of health benefits and harms, any explicit treatment of patient preferences, or any estimates of the cost implications of their recommendations, certainly not in comparison with alternative practices. Most also lack explicit assessments of the strength of the evidence behind their recommendations."[13] The committee endorsed a set of desirable attributes for guidelines, giving first priority to scientific validity and recommending careful documentation of the evidence and the process used. According to the committee's definition, a guideline is valid if it produces, in practice, "the health and cost outcomes projected" for it; the definition underscores the central role of the projections.[14]

Some attempts have already been made to develop better processes, and they offer valuable building blocks for the future. The Canadian Task Force on the Periodic Health Exam designed a rigorous system for evaluating medical evidence and rating the strength of recommendations based on it, which was used by the U.S. Preventive Services Task Force early in its deliberations.[15] The Office of Technology Assessment in the U.S. Congress routinely uses formal methods of evaluation, particularly cost-effectiveness analysis, to support its recommendations to Congress.[16] And the American College of Physicians has published a series of recommendations created through a process in which the guiding principles were that the recommendations should be based on evidence and on "an explicit understanding of the benefits, harms, and costs of screening to patients."[17]

An improved decisionmaking process needs built-in safeguards to ensure that all major aspects of a recommendation are considered. The burden placed on patients by falsely positive test results should be weighed along with the risk of missing disease; the side effects of treatment along with its life-saving potential; the problems posed by real-world laboratory quality, and failure to coordinate testing and treatment, along with the value of the test in research settings. The more factors considered, the more complicated the decisionmaking process becomes. Cost-effectiveness analysis and meta-analysis provide essential tools for establishing a decisionmaking framework and evaluating the elements that belong in it. If they were incorporated regularly into the decisionmaking process, they would improve it substantially. At the same time, regular use of these analytic tools would be the biggest impetus to their continued improvement.

Allocating Resources to Screening

While developers have a responsibility to estimate the benefits and costs of their recommendations, final decisions about resource allocation will be shared with policymakers at other levels—insurers, employers, and government officials. These payers have responsibility for insisting that resources actually be considered, not just estimated and ignored, in making screening policy. Resources claimed by screening tests are denied to other worthwhile purposes. Decisions about resource allocation should be based on benefits in relation to costs, not because dollars matter in and of themselves, but because they represent opportunities lost. When millions of dollars are spent on screening that yields little or no improvement in health, while medical services that could accomplish much more are not funded, the opportunity cost of that screening is high.

The estimates of costs and cost-effectiveness for screening for cervical cancer, prostate cancer, and high blood cholesterol show that there are major problems with the current allocation of medical resources in the United States, many in the form of decisions, such as how often to screen or what dosage of a drug to use, that do not appear to be of much consequence. The billions of dollars involved in these three screening tests alone are enough to finance a system of basic care for the poor and uninsured.[18] The money spent on screening and treating healthy adults for high blood cholesterol could finance a program of prenatal care for all low-income pregnant women. And funds that now go to screening for prostate cancer could be used instead to ensure that all children are properly immunized by age two.

These choices may be of only hypothetical interest to some, but they are real for any decisionmaker working with a fixed budget. Medicaid is a prime example. States are hard put to finance the demands on their Medicaid programs, even as Medicaid expenditures crowd out spending on other programs. The examples considered in this book suggest that Medicaid administrators may be able to make their budgets accomplish more by reallocating funds from some services to others. Overinvestments that result from current screening recommendations offer the opportunity to shift resources to other, more beneficial services, or to people who are not now covered at all.

In an attempt to stretch its Medicaid funds to cover all low-income people in the state, Oregon has proposed a plan based on setting priorities among services.[19] The priority-setting process ignores costs except when deciding how much of the list to cover. Screening tests, part of preventive services for adults, are ranked above hip replacements in this system, with no restrictions on how often the tests should be performed or for which adults. Pap smears every three or five years qualify as essential, but what about annual Pap smears? Are they really higher priority than hip replacements, which can restore elderly people's ability to get around on their own? The cost-effectiveness results for cervical cancer screening suggest that they may not be.

The cost-effectiveness analyses show clearly that the problem is not simply one of too much screening. Overinvestment exists side by side with underinvestment in the same test—both the Pap smear and screening for high blood cholesterol provide examples. The split exists in part because of the patchwork system of coverage in the United States, which gives some people, but not others, ready and convenient access to medical care. Those with access will get Pap smears and cholesterol tests often, more often than is a productive use of medical resources, while those without it may not get them at all. While individual programs like Medicaid may be able to improve the distribution of services within the program, the more important inequities are beyond their control.

Viewed in the context of the larger medical care system, these inequities show how the problems of cost and access in the United States are played out in terms of particular services. The solution to the larger and the smaller problems is the same: more for those who currently receive little, a bit less for those who currently receive a lot. A more equitable distribution of medical resources would be a more productive one as well, yielding a healthier nation for the same expenditure of resources.

Appendix: Details of the Estimates in Figure 5

The guesstimate of lives saved by radical prostatectomy is based on a statement by Patrick Walsh, prominent urologist and surgeon, that the death rate from prostate cancer in Sweden is 10 percent higher than that in the United States.[20] Treatment for later prostate cancer is agreed to be ineffective (see Chapter 3) so, if the difference in death rates reflects differences in treatment, it would have to be due entirely to the (unproven) benefit of radical prostatectomy for early cancers. If it is assumed that 25 percent of all prostate cancers are detected at an appropriate stage for surgery, then prostatectomy would have to reduce the death rate of these patients over ten years by 40 percent in order to produce an overall difference of 10 percent. The 25 percent assumption is reasonable—not all cancers are detected in time and, of those that appear to be on the basis of initial tests, half turn out to be too far advanced when surgery is actually performed—but the precise number was chosen arbitrarily to provide a clear and simple difference in lives saved by the U.S. approach.

The data in Tables 1 and 4 of the article about the Swedish study indicated that, in Sweden, virtually all of the patients whose disease progressed were treated. The article stated that hormonal treatment could be either drugs or orchidectomy (removal of the testicles), but did not state how often each was used. It was assumed that the surgical death rate for orchidectomy is the same as that for radical prostatectomy, between 1 and 2 percent. If this is true, there would be less than 0.2 of a death associated with orchidectomy. In light of the small number and the optimistic assumption made about the benefit of radical prostatectomy, this 0.2 of a death was ignored in the calculations.

To arrive at estimates of the number of years of treatment (or the number of years post-treatment), it was assumed that, except for the man who dies during the radical prostatectomy, those who die survive an average of five years. It was also assumed that, in Sweden, treatment begins an average of one year after the beginning of the study for those who die, and two years after for those who survive. About 20 percent of the men who did not show progression in Sweden were treated for local problems. The same assumptions were made about how soon their treatment started after the beginning of the study.

It was assumed that the numbers of deaths from other causes would be equal in both countries, and that, in Sweden, deaths from other causes are distributed proportionately across all men who do not die of prostate cancer, whether or not they experience progression.

Notes

1. Introduction

1. U.S. Preventive Services Task Force, *Guide to Clinical Preventive Services: An Assessment of the Effectiveness of 169 Interventions* (Baltimore: Williams and Wilkins, 1989).

2. Screening for Cervical Cancer

1. In 1948 the American Cancer Society convened a conference on methods of diagnosing cancer from cellular material that helped promote the use of the Pap test. J. Mostyn David, "Pap Tests Needed for Women of All Ages," *Postgraduate Medicine* 89 (January 1991): 27, 30.

2. Anne-Marie Foltz and Jennifer L. Kelsey, "The Annual Pap Test: A Dubious Policy Success," *Milbank Memorial Fund Quarterly/Health and Society* 56, no. 4 (1978): 426–62; National Cancer Institute, "New System for Reporting Pap Smears," press release, August 17, 1989.

3. For a description of the classification system in which the term *dysplasia* is replaced by the term *cervical intraepithelial lesion* (CIN), see Charlotte Muller, Jeanne Mandelblatt, Clyde B. Schechter, Elaine J. Power, Brigitte M. Duffy, and Judith L. Wagner, *The Costs and Effectiveness of Cervical Cancer Screening in Elderly Women* (Office of Technology Assessment, U.S. Congress, February 1990), pp. 3–4. In 1989 a

system separating abnormal results short of invasive cancer into two classes, low-grade and high-grade squamous intraepithelial lesions, was proposed by the National Cancer Institute. See National Cancer Institute Workshop, "The 1988 Bethesda System for Reporting Cervical/Vaginal Cytological Diagnoses," *Journal of the American Medical Association* 262 (August 18, 1989): 931–34.

4. Muller et al., *Costs and Effectiveness of Cervical Cancer Screening in Elderly Women*, pp. 16–17; Sally Squires, "The Importance of Pap Tests," *Washington Post Health*, July 24, 1990, p. WH9.

5. IARC Working Group on Evaluation of Cervical Cancer Screening Programmes, "Screening for Squamous Cervical Cancer: Duration of Low Risk after Negative Results of Cervical Cytology and Its Implication for Screening Policies," *British Medical Journal* 293 (September 13, 1986): 659–64.

6. The analysis was based primarily on the "case-control" method, which compares the screening histories of women who developed invasive cervical cancer ("cases") with women, matched for age, who did not ("controls"). The results showed that controls were more likely to have been screened (and treated for any abnormalities) than were cases, and that controls were screened more often. Some of the screening programs that contributed data to the study matched cases and controls for characteristics in addition to age, such as place of residence or marital status. IARC Working Group, "Screening for Squamous Cervical Cancer," p. 660 and Table 1.

7. Matt Clark, Mariana Gosnell, Mary Hager, and June Morrall, "Questions about the Pap Test," *Newsweek*, January 25, 1988, pp. 57–58.

8. The following organizations endorsed the recommendation: American Cancer Society, National Cancer Institute, American College of Obstetricians and Gynecologists, American

Medical Association, American Nurses Association, American Academy of Family Physicians, and American Medical Women's Association. See Gina Kolata, "Medical Groups Reach Compromise on Frequency of Giving Pap Tests," *New York Times*, January 7, 1988, p. B13; U.S. Preventive Services Task Force, *Guide to Clinical Preventive Services: An Assessment of the Effectiveness of 169 Interventions* (Baltimore: Williams and Wilkins, 1989), p. 58.

9. American Cancer Society, *Guidelines for the Cancer-Related Health Checkup: Recommendations and Rationale* (New York: American Cancer Society, 1980).

10. Foltz and Kelsey, "The Annual Pap Test."

11. See Clark et al., "Questions about the Pap Test," p. 57; "How Electronic Eyes Speed Up Pap Tests," *Business Week*, November 27, 1989, p. 99; Robin Marantz Henig, "Is the Pap Test Valid?" *New York Times Magazine*, May 28, 1989, p. 37; Squires, "Importance of Pap Tests," p. WH9; and U.S. Preventive Services Task Force, *Guide to Clinical Preventive Services*, p. 57. The test results in these cases are termed "false negatives" because they show falsely that the woman does not have disease.

12. IARC Working Group, "Screening for Squamous Cervical Cancer."

13. An Australian study of cancers that occurred within three years of a negative Pap test found that only 12 percent of the tests were based on an adequate sample of cervical cells. See Heather Mitchell, Gabriele Medley, and Graham Giles, "Cervical Cancers Diagnosed after Negative Results on Cervical Cytology: Perspective in the 1980s," *British Medical Journal* 300 (June 23, 1990): 1622–26.

14. David M. Eddy, "Screening for Cervical Cancer," *Annals of Internal Medicine* 113 (August 1, 1990): 224.

15. She is unlikely to be aware of two others. According to an article in *Working Woman*, the timing of the test can improve

its accuracy. The test should be scheduled when there is no menstrual bleeding and at least twenty-four hours after intercourse or douching. No information is presented, however, to suggest how much this improves test accuracy. Sy Montgomery, "Smart Planning for the Pap Smear," *Working Woman*, April 1989, p. 160. A woman can also request a copy of the test report and if the lab uses the Bethesda System of reporting can learn from it whether the sample was adequate. If it was not, her options once again reduce to having another test.

16. IARC data for British Columbia and Manitoba support the idea that repeat tests were independent in those two Canadian provinces. See IARC Working Group, "Screening for Squamous Cervical Cancer," p. 662.

17. More precisely, only 0.75 of the cases will remain undetected.

18. Kolata, "Medical Groups Reach Compromise"; Stanley A. Gall, "Pap Smears—Do Them Right and Every Year—Forever!" *Postgraduate Medicine* 85 (May 1, 1989): 235–39.

19. Henig, "Is the Pap Test Valid?" p. 38.

20. Muller et al., *Costs and Effects of Cervical Cancer Screening in Elderly Women*, p. 9; Eddy, "Screening for Cervical Cancer," p. 214; Gall, "Pap Smears," p. 237; Clark et al., "Questions about the Pap Test," p. 58.

21. Henig, "Is the Pap Test Valid?"

22. Muller et al., *Costs and Effectiveness of Cervical Cancer Screening in Elderly Women*, p. 23.

23. McCormick is one of the few writers, even in the medical literature, to draw attention to the high lifetime risk of a false positive test result. See James S. McCormick, "Cervical Smears: A Questionable Practice?" *Lancet* 2, no. 8656 (July 22, 1989): 207–9.

24. U.S. Preventive Services Task Force, *Guide to Clinical Preventive Services*, p. 57.

25. Eddy, "Screening for Cervical Cancer."

26. In 1990, in the wake of articles in the *Wall Street Journal* about the inaccuracy of Pap smears, the federal government proposed new rules to improve test accuracy in labs participating in the Medicare and Medicaid programs. See Kenneth H. Bacon, "Rules Set to Improve Pap Smears," *Wall Street Journal,* March 12, 1990, p. B1. The "Bethesda System" of nomenclature, proposed in 1988, is also intended to increase the accuracy of test results by improving communication between labs and doctors. (See National Cancer Institute Workshop, "The 1988 Bethesda System.") In addition, two systems for using computers to help with the tedious and difficult work of reading slides are under development. See Judith Randal, "Better, More Accurate Pap Tests Being Designed," *Washington Post,* February 27, 1990, p. WH5; and Gregory Crouch, "Biomed Firms Race to Improve Pap Smear Tests," *Los Angeles Times,* April 15, 1990, pp. D1, D8.

27. McCormick, "Cervical Smears: A Questionable Practice?"

28. D. K. Ohrt, "The Intraepithelial Lesion: A Spectrum of Problems," *Journal of the American Medical Association* 262, no. 7 (August 18, 1989): 944–45.

29. Muller et al., *Costs and Effectiveness of Cervical Cancer Screening in Elderly Women,* pp. 11–12.

30. Foltz and Kelsey, "The Annual Pap Test," p. 435; Astrid Fletcher, "Screening for Cancer of the Cervix in Elderly Women," *Lancet* 335 (January 13, 1990): 98.

31. Eddy, "Screening for Cervical Cancer," Table 3.

32. *Ibid.,* p. 223.

33. David Eddy, cited in Kolata, "Medical Groups Reach Compromise." The same estimates appear in Clark et al., "Questions about the Pap Test." Eddy's estimate of $75 for the cost of the test and the physician's visit seems high for 1985, the year he used, but it may be closer to the true average in 1993. Thus his estimate of the total cost of screening may be approximately right for the early 1990s.

34. The dollar figures are for the late 1980s. Ohrt, "The Intraepithelial Lesion: A Spectrum of Problems."

35. The calculations for Eddy's model were carried out for a single woman as she aged, using probabilities of various outcomes for each age taken from the IARC study and other relevant literature. See Eddy, "Screening for Cervical Cancer," esp. Table 3 and the appendix on pp. 224–25. The results could thus be expressed in terms of the average number of days of life saved and the related costs for one woman. The published numbers, presented in Figure 2 of this chapter, were derived by dividing the days of life saved by the dollar cost (both discounted at 5 percent) to find the cost per year of life saved. In effect, the results for one woman were multiplied by the number of women who must be screened to produce one year of life.

36. Eddy, "Screening for Cervical Cancer." Eddy uses the following costs based on data for 1985: the initial test and physician's visit, $75; workup of a false positive, $150; treatment of carcinoma in situ, and of abnormalities that would have regressed on their own, $5,641; treatment of invasive cervical cancer—$11,600 for Stage I, $16,891 for Stages II and III, and $18,587 for Stage IV; terminal care for a patient dying of cervical cancer, $22,150.

37. Jonathon T. Edelson, Milton C. Weinstein, Anna N. A. Tosteson, Larry Williams, Thomas H. Lee, and Lee Goldman, "Long-Term Cost-Effectiveness of Various Initial Monotherapies for Mild to Moderate Hypertension," *Journal of the American Medical Association* 263 (January 19, 1990): 407–13; Louise B. Russell, "Some of the Tough Decisions Required by a National Health Plan," *Science* 246 (November 17, 1989): 892–96.

38. P. B. S. Silcocks and S. M. Moss, "Rapidly Progressive Cervical Cancer: Is It a Real Problem?" *British Journal of Obstetrics and Gynaecology* 95 (November 1988): 1111–16.

39. Mitchell, Medley, and Giles, "Cervical Cancers Diagnosed after Negative Results on Cervical Cytology."

40. Jeanne S. Mandelblatt and Marianne C. Fahs, "The Cost-Effectiveness of Cervical Cancer Screening for Low-Income Elderly Women," *Journal of the American Medical Association* 261 (April 22/29, 1988): 2409–13.

41. R. Ellman, "Problems of Follow-Up for Abnormal Cervical Smears: Discussion Paper," *Journal of the Royal Society of Medicine* 83 (February 1990), pp. 94–95.

3. Screening for Prostate Cancer

1. *Cancer Facts and Figures, 1991* (Atlanta: American Cancer Society, 1991). Don Dunn, "Prostate Cancer: How to Thwart a Killer," *Business Week*, March 16, 1992, pp. 132–33.

2. "Choices for Prostate Cancer Treatment," *USA Today*, February 1988, p. 5; Joanne Silberner, "Conquering Prostate Cancer," *U.S. News and World Report*, July 10, 1989, pp. 55–57. Dunn, "Prostate Cancer: How to Thwart a Killer."

3. Robert A. Badalament and Joseph R. Drago, "Prostate Cancer," *Disease-a-Month* (April 1991): 234–38.

4. Larry Thompson, "Prostate Cancer and Potency," *Washington Post*, June 23, 1987, p. HE6a. Badalament and Drago, "Prostate Cancer," pp. 244–47.

5. Dunn, "Prostate Cancer: How to Thwart a Killer," p. 132.

6. William J. Catalona, Deborah S. Smith, Timothy L. Ratliff, Kathy M. Dodds, Douglas E. Coplen, Jerry J.J. Yuan, John A. Petros, and Gerald L. Andriole, "Measurement of Prostate-Specific Antigen in Serum as a Screening Test for Prostate Cancer," *New England Journal of Medicine* 324 (April 25, 1991): 1156–61.

7. Ron Winslow, "New Blood Test Found to Detect Prostate Cancer," *Wall Street Journal*, April 25, 1991, p. B1; "Prostate Cancer: Sounding an Early Alarm," *Business Week*, May

6, 1991, p. 130; "Unmasking a Stealthy Cancer," *Time,* May 6, 1991, p. 45. Dunn, "Prostate Cancer: How to Thwart a Killer."

8. Winslow, "New Blood Test."

9. "Unmasking a Stealthy Cancer."

10. U.S. Preventive Services Task Force, *Guide to Clinical Preventive Services: An Assessment of the Effectiveness of 169 Interventions* (Baltimore: Williams and Wilkins, 1989), p. 64. The statement is based on D. P. Byar, D. K. Corle, and the Veterans Administration Cooperative Urological Research Group, "VACURG Randomized Trial of Radical Prostatectomy for Stages I and II Prostate Cancer," *Urology* 17, supp. 4 (April 1981), pp. 7–11.

11. Gary D. Friedman, Robert A. Hiatt, Charles P. Quesenberry, Jr., and Joseph V. Selby, "Case-Control Study of Screening for Prostatic Cancer by Digital Rectal Examinations," *Lancet* 337 (June 22, 1991): 1526–29.

12. Gerald W. Chodak, in a letter published together with the article by Frank Hinman, Jr., "Screening for Prostatic Carcinoma," *Journal of Urology* 145 (January 1991): 126–30.

13. Badalament and Drago, "Prostate Cancer," p. 209.

14. L. M. Franks, "Latent Carcinoma of the Prostate," *Journal of Pathology and Bacteriology* 68 (1954), pp. 603–16.

15. Badalament and Drago, "Prostate Cancer," p. 219; Gerald W. Chodak, Paul Keller, and Harry W. Schoenberg, "Assessment of Screening for Prostate Cancer Using the Digital Rectal Examination," *Journal of Urology* 141 (May 1989), p. 1138; Fred Lee, Soren T. Torp-Pedersen, Peter J. Littrup, and Richard D. McLeary, "Is Ultrasound of the Prostate Indicated for Screening Purposes? An Affirmative View," *Journal of Family Practice* 27 (1988): 521.

16. For definitions and discussions of lead-time bias and the other biases discussed in this chapter, see U.S. Preventive Services Task Force, *Guide to Clinical Preventive Services,* p. xxxii;

Philip C. Prorok, Robert J. Connor, and Stuart G. Baker, "Statistical Considerations in Cancer Screening Programs," *Urologic Clinics of North America* 17 (November 1990): 699–708; Charlotte Muller, Jeanne Mandelblatt, Clyde B. Schechter, Elaine J. Power, Brigitte M. Duffy, and Judith L. Wagner, *Costs and Effectiveness of Cervical Cancer Screening in Elderly Women* (U.S. Congress, Office of Technology Assessment, February 1990), p. 25; and Gerald W. Chodak, "Early Detection and Screening for Prostatic Cancer," *Urology* 34, supp. 4 (October 1989): 11.

17. Prorok, Connor, and Baker, "Statistical Considerations in Cancer Screening Programs."

18. The usual practice is to focus on deaths from the disease that screening (or treatment) is expected to influence. To guard against the possibility of adverse effects on other conditions, however, trials should include more comprehensive endpoints, such as deaths from all causes. The case of high blood cholesterol, discussed in the next chapter, provides a telling example.

19. Hinman, "Screening for Prostatic Carcinoma"; Chodak, Keller, and Schoenberg, "Assessment of Screening for Prostate Cancer Using the Digital Rectal Examination," p. 1138.

20. Linda Schwab, "Experts Sharply Divided on Prostate Cancer Screening," *Journal of the National Cancer Institute* 83 (April 17, 1991): 535–36; National Cancer Institute, "DCPC Project Review" and "PLCO Concept," Bethesda, Md., January 1991.

21. See Byar, Corle, and the Veterans Administration Cooperative Urological Research Group, "VACURG Randomized Trial of Radical Prostatectomy"; and Peder H. Graversen, Knud T. Nielsen, Thomas C. Gasser, Donald K. Corle, and Paul O. Madsen, "Radical Prostatectomy Versus Expectant Primary Treatment in Stages I and II Prostatic Cancer: A Fifteen-Year Follow-up," *Urology* 36 (December 1990):

493–98. Methods of screening were not part of the trial and randomization helped to insure that, whatever the nature of the cancer and however it was discovered, the patient's assignment to a treatment group would not be influenced. Thus survival is an acceptable measure of outcome in a study of this kind because there is no reason to expect the natural history of cancers in one group to differ from that of cancers in the other, except as a result of the treatment.

22. Case-control methods are attracting increasing interest for the evaluation of screening; see Anthony B. Miller, "Screening for Cancer: State of the Art and Prospects for the Future," *World Journal of Surgery* 13 (January–February 1989): 79. The method was described briefly in note 6, Chapter 2. For this kind of study, men who died of prostate cancer ("cases") would be compared with a matched group of men who did not ("controls") to see whether there were differences in the frequency with which the two groups were screened. If cases were screened significantly less often than controls, that suggests that screening is beneficial. Case-control studies have an advantage over randomized controlled trials—they can use historical ("retrospective") data and produce useful results from much smaller samples. It is, however, difficult to be sure that the matching process produces two groups that are alike in every way except their screening history. Friedman and his colleagues used this method in their study of the digital rectal exam (see "Case-Control Study of Screening for Prostatic Cancer by Digital Rectal Examinations"); they used the development of metastatic prostate cancer as the endpoint since it is known that current treatment is largely ineffective for prostate cancer that has metastasized.

23. Hinman, "Screening for Prostatic Carcinoma"; David J. Chadwick, Terry Kemple, J. Peter Astley, Angus G. MacIver, David A. Gillatt, Paul Abrams, and J. Clive Gingell, "Pilot Study of Screening for Prostate Cancer in General Practice," *Lancet* 338 (September 7, 1991): 613–16.

24. U.S. Preventive Services Task Force, *Guide to Clinical Preventive Services*, p. 63.

25. Chodak, Keller, and Schoenberg, "Assessment of Screening for Prostate Cancer Using the Digital Rectal Examination."

26. U.S. Preventive Services Task Force, *Guide to Clinical Preventive Services*, p. 63; Hinman, "Screening for Prostatic Carcinoma," p. 126.

27. Lee et al., "Is Ultrasound of the Prostate Indicated for Screening Purposes?" Table 2, p. 523; Hinman, "Screening for Prostatic Carcinoma," pp. 126–27; U.S. Preventive Services Task Force, *Guide to Clinical Preventive Services*, p. 64.

28. Hinman, "Screening for Prostatic Carcinoma," p. 127.

29. Joseph E. Oesterling, "Prostate Specific Antigen: A Critical Assessment of the Most Useful Tumor Marker for Adenocarcinoma of the Prostate," *Journal of Urology* 145 (May 1991): 907–23.

30. These are the units used in Catalona et al., "Measurement of Prostate-Specific Antigen in Serum as a Screening Test for Prostate Cancer." Most of the literature uses different but equivalent terminology: 4 ng/ml (nanograms per milliliter).

31. Oesterling, "Prostate Specific Antigen," p. 920.

32. Hinman, "Screening for Prostatic Carcinoma," p. 127; Oesterling, "Prostate Specific Antigen," p. 913.

33. Oesterling, "Prostate Specific Antigen," p. 913.

34. Catalona et al., "Measurement of Prostate-Specific Antigen in Serum as a Screening Test for Prostate Cancer."

35. In the National Cancer Institute trial, the screening protocol for prostate cancer is based on an annual digital rectal exam and a PSA blood test for each man. If both tests are positive, a biopsy will be taken. If one of the two is positive, the prostate will be imaged by ultrasound and a biopsy taken if it shows a suspicious area. If both tests are negative, nothing

further will be done and the man returns for another screen the next year. National Cancer Institute, "PLCO Concept," p. 10.

36. U.S. Preventive Services Task Force, *Guide to Clinical Preventive Services*, pp. 63–65.

37. There is not much point in analyzing the cost-effectiveness of interventions whose effectiveness has not been established. The only published cost-effectiveness analysis of screening for prostate cancer is a kind of "what-if" exercise. For example, in the absence of any evidence for the effectiveness of screening or surgery, the authors assumed that radical prostatectomy is 100 percent effective in curing early-stage prostate cancer. Richard R. Love and Dennis G. Fryback, with the assistance of Steven R. Kimbrough, "A Cost-Effectiveness Analysis of Screening for Carcinoma of the Prostate by Digital Examination," *Medical Decision Making* 5 (1986): 263–78.

38. Badalament and Drago, "Prostate Cancer," pp. 217–18; Hinman, "Screening for Prostatic Carcinoma," p. 128.

39. Catalona et al., "Measurement of Prostate-Specific Antigen in Serum as a Screening Test for Prostate Cancer," p. 1157.

40. Chadwick et al., "Pilot Study of Screening for Prostate Cancer in General Practice," p. 615; Badalament and Drago, "Prostate Cancer," pp. 232–33.

41. Chodak, "Early Detection and Screening for Prostatic Cancer."

42. Don Colburn, "The Prostate and Its Problems," *Washington Post*, December 23, 1986, p. HE7A.

43. Edmund J. Graves, "1990 Summary: National Hospital Discharge Survey" (U.S. Department of Health and Human Services, National Center for Health Statistics, Advance Data no. 210, February 18, 1992), Table 7.

44. Colburn, "The Prostate and Its Problems"; Lawrence K. Altman, "President Is Well after Operation to Ease Prostate," *New York Times*, January 6, 1987, p. A14.

45. If early detection and treatment are effective, there may be savings in treatment costs to offset some of these costs.

46. Martin L. Brown, Arnold L. Potosky, Grey B. Thompson, and Larry G. Kessler, "The Knowledge and Use of Screening Tests for Colorectal and Prostate Cancer: Data from the 1987 National Health Interview Survey," *Preventive Medicine* 19 (1990): 562–74. In 1987, 20 percent of men reported having had a digital rectal exam in the last year. Since some of them undoubtedly are examined less often than annually, this is a high estimate of the percent who meet the ACS guideline.

47. Paul Chang and Gerald W. Friedland, "The Role of Imaging in Screening for Prostate Cancer: A Decision Analysis Perspective," *Investigative Radiology* 25 (May 1990): 595; Gerald W. Chodak and Harry W. Schoenberg, "Progress and Problems in Screening for Carcinoma of the Prostate," *World Journal of Surgery* 13 (January-February 1989): 63.

48. See the appendix to Chapter 3 for details.

49. Jane E. Brody, "Nationwide Tests Set for Prostate Cancer, But Doubts Surface," *New York Times*, September 20, 1992, pp. 1, 30.

50. Catalona et al., "Measurement of Prostate-Specific Antigen in Serum as a Screening Test for Prostate Cancer."

51. The cost per visit comes from Lee et al., "Is Ultrasound of the Prostate Indicated for Screening Purposes?" and the cost of the test is taken from "Unmasking a Stealthy Cancer," *Time*, May 6, 1991, p. 45. I checked the cost of the test against the charges of two labs that serve hospitals affiliated with the University of Medicine and Dentistry of New Jersey (in New Brunswick, New Jersey) and one lab that serves nearby physicians' offices. Those charges were $91, $72, and $35, respectively, so $50 seems like a reasonable estimate of the average.

52. Lee et al., "Is Ultrasound of the Prostate Indicated for Screening Purposes?" One physicians' group in central New Jersey charges $1,050 for a biopsy.

4. Screening for High Blood Cholesterol

1. For a description of the defining features of a randomized controlled trial, see Chapter 3.

2. Lipid Research Clinics Program, "The Lipid Research Clinics Coronary Primary Prevention Trial Results, II: The Relationship of Reduction in Incidence of Coronary Heart Disease to Cholesterol Lowering," *Journal of the American Medical Association* 251 (January 20, 1984): 365–74. In fact, an earlier trial—known as the World Health Organization trial—demonstrated that lowering blood cholesterol lowered the incidence of heart attacks, but the group whose cholesterol was lowered by drugs suffered more deaths overall than the control group, an effect which was attributed to Clofibrate, the particular drug used in the trial. See M. F. Oliver, J. A. Heady, J. N. Morris, and J. Cooper, "A Co-operative Trial in the Primary Prevention of Ischaemic Heart Disease Using Clofibrate: Report from the Committee of Principal Investigators," *British Heart Journal* 40 (1978): 1069–118.

3. National Cholesterol Education Program, *High Blood Cholesterol in Adults: Report of the Expert Panel on Detection, Evaluation, and Treatment* (Bethesda, Md.: National Institutes of Health, U.S. Department of Health and Human Services), January 1988. The report was also published in the *Archives of Internal Medicine*. See "Report of the National Cholesterol Education Program Expert Panel on Detection, Evaluation, and Treatment of High Blood Cholesterol in Adults," *Archives of Internal Medicine* 148 (January 1988): 36–69.

4. U.S. Bureau of the Census, *Statistical Abstract of the United States 1991*, 111th ed. (Washington, D.C., 1991), Table 12.

5. National Cholesterol Education Program, *High Blood Cholesterol in Adults*, appendix I.

6. Christopher Sempos, Robinson Fulwood, Carol Haines, Margaret Carroll, Robert Anda, David F. Williamson, Patrick

Remington, and James Cleeman, "The Prevalence of High Blood Cholesterol Levels among Adults in the United States," *Journal of the American Medical Association* 262 (July 7, 1989): 45–52.

7. Beth Schucker, Janet T. Wittes, Nancy C. Santanello, Stephen J. Weber, Daniel McGoldrick, Karen Donato, Alan Levy, and Basil M. Rifkind, "Change in Cholesterol Awareness and Action: Results from National Physician and Public Surveys," *Archives of Internal Medicine* 151 (April 1991): 666.

8. Marian Burros, "Eating Well," *New York Times*, January 13, 1988, p. C4.

9. Thomas J. Moore, "The Cholesterol Myth," *Atlantic*, September 1989, pp. 37–70.

10. Moore was not the first to make the point in the general media, but his article was the first to gain widespread attention. For example, Hanauer said many of the same things very briefly in an op-ed piece. See Lonnie B. Hanauer, "Cholesterol Phobia," *New York Times*, June 13, 1988, p. A19.

11. Gina Kolata, "Major Study Aims to Learn Who Should Lower Cholesterol," *New York Times*, September 26, 1989, pp. C1, C11.

12. "Doubts about the Cholesterol Crusade," *New York Times*, September 14, 1989, p. A28.

13. Andrew Purvis, "Don't Go Back to Butter," *Time*, October, 1989, p. 108. John Pekkanen, "New Questions about Cholesterol," *Reader's Digest*, April 1990, pp. 103–8. "Forget about Cholesterol?" *Consumer Reports*, March 1990, pp. 152–57.

14. Matthew F. Muldoon, Stephen B. Manuck, and Karen A. Matthews, "Lowering Cholesterol Concentrations and Mortality: A Quantitative Review of Primary Prevention Trials," *British Medical Journal* 301 (August 11, 1990): 309–14. The authors used meta-analytical techniques to make judgments

about the statistical validity of their generalizations across the six trials.

15. The six trials were the Helsinki Heart Study of men ages forty to fifty-five, which excluded anyone with evidence of heart disease or insulin-dependent diabetes; the Lipid Research Clinics trial of men thirty-five to fifty-nine, which excluded those with heart disease, diabetes, or hypertension; the Colestipol-Upjohn study of adults, which excluded those with liver, kidney, or thyroid disease; the World Health Organization (WHO) study of men thirty to fifty-nine, which excluded those with heart disease, diabetes, or hypertension; the Minnesota Coronary Survey of adults in mental hospitals, which had no health restrictions on enrollment; and the Los Angeles Veterans Administration study of men over age fifty-five, which excluded those with diabetes, alcohol abuse, or serious illness of any kind.

16. Salim Yusuf applied meta-analysis to thirty-two randomized controlled trials that collectively enrolled more than 42,000 people. The results are briefly summarized in David Jacobs, Henry Blackburn, Millicent Higgins, et al., "Report of the Conference on Low Blood Cholesterol: Mortality Associations," *Circulation* 86 (September 1992): 1055. Ingar Holme, who also combined trials in healthy men with those in heart-attack patients, found an initial adverse effect of treatment (in terms of total deaths) that was gradually overcome, as cholesterol was further reduced, by a reduction in deaths from heart disease. Holme estimated that total deaths would begin to decline once blood cholesterol had been reduced by at least 8 or 9 percent. But since the trend was stronger in the trials that enrolled heart-attack patients, the overall result may have been entirely due to those trials. See Ingar Holme, "An Analysis of Randomized Trials Evaluating the Effect of Cholesterol Reduction on Total Mortality and Coronary Heart Disease Incidence," *Circulation* 82 (December 1990): 1916–24.

17. Jacobs et al., "Report of the Conference on Low Blood Cholesterol: Mortality Associations," p. 1056.

18. Stephen B. Hulley, Judith M. B. Walsh, and Thomas B. Newman, "Health Policy on Blood Cholesterol: Time to Change Directions," *Circulation* 86 (September 1992): 1027.

19. National Cholesterol Education Program, *High Blood Cholesterol in Adults*, p. 15.

20. Paul L. Canner, Kenneth G. Berge, Nanette K. Wenger, Jeremiah Stamler, Lawrence Friedman, Ronald J. Prineas, and William Friedewald for the Coronary Drug Project Research Group, "Fifteen-Year Mortality in Coronary Drug Project Patients: Long-Term Benefit with Niacin," *Journal of the American College of Cardiology* 8 (December 1986): 1245–55.

21. Jacques E. Rossouw, Barry Lewis, and Basil M. Rifkind, "The Value of Lowering Cholesterol after Myocardial Infarction," *New England Journal of Medicine* 323 (October 18, 1990): 1112–19, esp. Table 1. The authors described their results as based on "eight secondary prevention trials" (p. 1114), but strictly speaking, there were six trials, two of which tested two different therapies each; thus there were six trials and eight therapies (diet or drugs).

22. Many of the arguments in favor of cholesterol screening are stated in Rossouw, Lewis, and Rifkind, "The Value of Lowering Cholesterol after Myocardial Infarction," while many of the criticisms are presented in the report by the Toronto Working Group on Cholesterol Policy (C. David Naylor, Antoni Basinski, John W. Frank, and Michael M. Rachlis), *Asymptomatic Hypercholesterolemia: A Clinical Policy Review*, published as a special issue of the *Journal of Clinical Epidemiology* 43, no. 10 (1990), esp. chap. 3.

23. William B. Kannel, William P. Castelli, and Tavia Gordon, "Cholesterol in the Prediction of Atherosclerotic Disease," *Annals of Internal Medicine* 90 (January 1979): 85–91.

24. National Cholesterol Education Program, *High Blood Cholesterol in Adults*, p. 28.

25. Alan M. Garber, Benjamin Littenberg, Harold C. Sox, Jr., Michael E. Gluck, Judith L. Wagner, and Brigitte M. Duffy, *Costs and Effectiveness of Cholesterol Screening in the Elderly* (Washington, D.C.: Office of Technology Assessment, U.S. Congress, April 1989).

26. Dr. Thomas N. James in Gina Kolata, "Major Study Aims to Learn Who Should Lower Cholesterol."

27. National Cholesterol Education Program, *High Blood Cholesterol in Adults*, p. 46.

28. "NCEP Releases Report on Cholesterol in Children," *American Family Physician* 43 (June 1991): 2263–64. American Academy of Pediatrics, "Statement on Cholesterol," *Pediatrics* 90 (September 1992): 469–73.

29. Ken Resnicow, Jane Morley-Kotchen, and Ernst Wynder, "Plasma Cholesterol Levels of 6585 Children in the United States: Results of the Know Your Body Screening in Five States," *Pediatrics* 84 (December 1989): 969–76. "New Studies Fuel Controversy over Universal Cholesterol Screening during Childhood," *Journal of the American Medical Association* 261 (February 10, 1989): 814. Steven Findlay, "Pondering the Ice-Cream Question," *U.S. News and World Report*, February 15, 1988, p. 78.

30. American Academy of Pediatrics, "Statement on Cholesterol," p. 470.

31. Ronald M. Lauer and William R. Clarke, "Use of Cholesterol Measurement in Childhood for the Prediction of Adult Hypercholesterolemia: The Muscatine Study," *Journal of the American Medical Association* 264 (December 19, 1990): 3034–38.

32. Thomas B. Newman, Warren S. Browner, and Stephen B. Hulley, "The Case against Childhood Cholesterol Screen-

ing," *Journal of the American Medical Association* 264 (December 19, 1990): 3039–43. C. D. Naylor, "Dyslipidaemias and the Primary Prevention of Coronary Heart Disease: Reflections on Some Unresolved Policy Issues," chap. 23 in Phil Gold, Steven Grover, and Daniel A.K. Roncari, eds., *Cholesterol and Coronary Heart Disease: The Great Debate. Proceedings of an International Conference* (Park Ridge, N.J.: Parthenon Publishing Group, 1992), pp. 401–30.

33. Newman et al., "The Case against Childhood Cholesterol Screening."

34. "NCEP Releases Report on Cholesterol in Children."

35. Newman et al., "The Case against Childhood Cholesterol Screening," p. 3041.

36. Toronto Working Group on Cholesterol Policy, *Asymptomatic Hypercholesterolemia*, pp. 1078–79. Garber et al., *Costs and Effectiveness of Cholesterol Screening in the Elderly*, p. 20.

37. The standard deviation for the distribution of an individual's test values is typically 15 to 20 mg/dl. Toronto Working Group on Cholesterol Policy, *Asymptomatic Hypercholesterolemia*, p. 1078. For an individual with a true cholesterol level of 210 and a standard deviation of 15, 95 tests out of 100 would fall between 180 and 240.

38. National Cholesterol Education Program, *High Blood Cholesterol in Adults*, p. 21.

39. Garber et al., *Costs and Effectiveness of Cholesterol Screening in the Elderly*, p. 19.

40. The results of this study are reported in Garber et al., *Costs and Effectiveness of Cholesterol Screening in the Elderly*, p. 21; Toronto Working Group on Cholesterol Policy, *Asymptomatic Hypercholesterolemia*, p. 1079; and Newman et al., "The Case against Childhood Cholesterol Screening," p. 3040.

41. Garber et al., *Costs and Effectiveness of Cholesterol Screening in the Elderly*, p. 22. Toronto Working Group on Cholesterol Policy, *Asymptomatic Hypercholesterolemia*, p. 1080.

42. Les Irwig, Paul Glasziou, Andrew Wilson, and Petra Macaskill, "Estimating an Individual's True Cholesterol Level and Response to Intervention," *Journal of the American Medical Association* 266 (September 25, 1991): 1678–85. See also S. G. Thompson and S. J. Pocock, "The Variability of Serum Cholesterol Measurements: Implications for Screening and Monitoring," *Journal of Clinical Epidemiology* 43 (1990): 783–89.

43. William C. Taylor, Theodore M. Pass, Donald S. Shepard, and Anthony L. Komaroff, "Cholesterol Reduction and Life Expectancy: A Model Incorporating Multiple Risk Factors," *Annals of Internal Medicine* 106 (April 1987): 605–14.

44. The reductions were chosen to match the range of results from the Multiple Risk Factor Intervention Trial (MRFIT), in which diet was one of several interventions aimed at preventing heart disease. The average reduction in cholesterol for the intervention group was 6.7 percent, while the worst subgroup achieved only a 3 percent reduction and the best a 20 percent reduction. It is, however, highly unlikely that diet could reduce cholesterol by 20 percent for the average person—average reductions this large have only been achieved in experiments carried out in institutions. See Alan M. Garber and Judith L. Wagner, "Practice Guidelines and Cholesterol Policy," *Health Affairs* 10 (Summer 1991): 52–66.

45. Toronto Working Group on Cholesterol Policy, *Asymptomatic Hypercholesterolemia*, p. 1074. Clofibrate is rarely used since clinical trials showed that it increased overall mortality.

46. Murray Krahn, C. David Naylor, Antoni S. Basinski, and Allan S. Detsky, "Comparison of an Aggressive (U.S.) and Less Aggressive (Canadian) Policy for Cholesterol Screening

and Treatment," *Annals of Internal Medicine* 115 (August 15, 1991): 248–55.

47. Garber and Wagner, "Practice Guidelines and Cholesterol Policy."

48. Garber and Wagner also present estimates based on the assumption that LDL cholesterol is reduced 15 percent by diet alone. They note that average reductions of 15 percent have been achieved only in studies of people in institutions. Studies of people in the community have achieved reductions of less than 10 percent with diet.

49. William C. Taylor, Theodore M. Pass, Donald S. Shepard, and Anthony L. Komaroff, "Cost Effectiveness of Cholesterol Reduction for the Primary Prevention of Coronary Heart Disease in Men," in Richard B. Goldbloom and Robert S. Lawrence, eds., *Preventing Disease: Beyond the Rhetoric* (New York: Springer-Verlag, 1990), pp. 437–41. In addition to cholesterol determinations and other lab tests, the program involves two visits to a physician and ten to a dietitian during the first year, and one physician visit and three visits to a dietitian during all subsequent years.

50. Lee Goldman, Milton C. Weinstein, Paula A. Goldman, and Lawrence W. Williams, "Cost-Effectiveness of HMG-CoA Reductase Inhibition for Primary and Secondary Prevention of Coronary Heart Disease," *Journal of the American Medical Association* 265 (March 6, 1991): 1145–51. For the purposes of the analysis, healthy people are those who have no evidence of heart disease at the time they are screened for high cholesterol.

51. Toronto Working Group on Cholesterol Policy, *Asymptomatic Hypercholesterolemia*, p. 1062.

52. National Cholesterol Education Program, *High Blood Cholesterol in Adults*, p. 7. Toronto Working Group on Cholesterol Policy, *Asymptomatic Hypercholesterolemia*, chaps. 5 and 8. Allan S. Brett, "Treating Hypercholesterolemia: How

Should Physicians Interpret the Published Data for Patients?''
and Alexander Leaf, ''Management of Hypercholesterolemia: Are Preventive Interventions Advisable?'' both in *New
England Journal of Medicine* 321 (September 7, 1989):
676–80 and 680–84.

53. The executive summary was published in the *Archives of
Internal Medicine* and the full report in *Circulation*, both in
the same month. See National Cholesterol Education Program, ''Report of the Expert Panel on Population Strategies
for Blood Cholesterol Reduction: Executive Summary,'' *Archives of Internal Medicine* 151 (June 1991): 1071–84, and
''Report of the Expert Panel on Population Strategies for
Blood Cholesterol Reduction: A Statement from the National
Cholesterol Education Program, National Heart, Lung, and
Blood Institute, National Institutes of Health,'' special issue
of *Circulation* 83 (June 1991): 2154–232.

54. Toronto Working Group on Cholesterol Policy, *Asymptomatic Hypercholesterolemia*, p. 1037.

55. David Jacobs et al., ''Report of the Conference on Low Blood
Cholesterol: Mortality Associations.''

56. The Framingham Study, however, has not shown a family
history to be a factor in death from heart disease once other
risk factors have been taken into account. William C. Taylor,
personal communication.

57. The right decision is even less clear in light of a recent report
that studies that have found no effect of cholesterol-lowering
on deaths from heart disease have been ignored by those
writing on the subject. When these studies are taken into
account, the author concludes that lowering blood cholesterol ''is unlikely to prevent coronary heart disease.'' U.
Ravnskov, ''Cholesterol-Lowering Trials in Coronary Heart
Disease: Frequency of Citation and Outcome,'' *British Medical Journal* 305 (July 4, 1992): 15–19.

58. Stephen B. Hulley et al., ''Health Policy on Blood Cholesterol: Time to Change Directions.''

5. Conclusions

1. Population figures are for 1990 and are taken from the Bureau of the Census, *Statistical Abstract of the United States 1991*, 111th ed. (Washington, D.C., 1991), pp. 13 and 16.

2. Steven Findlay, "Pondering the Ice-Cream Question," *U.S. News and World Report*, February 15, 1988, p. 78.

3. Again, the exception to this statement is people who have already suffered heart attacks. In this group, where most deaths are from heart disease, studies show that cholesterol reduction probably does lengthen life.

4. From the Centers for Disease Control, "Regulations for Implementing Clinical Laboratory Improvement Amendments of 1988: A Summary," *Journal of the American Medical Association* 267 (April 1, 1992): 1725–27, 1731–34.

5. "Clinical Laboratory Improvement Amendments Finally May Go into Effect September 1," *Journal of the American Medical Association* 267 (March 18, 1992): 1441.

6. Centers for Disease Control, "Regulations for Implementing Clinical Laboratory Improvement Amendments of 1988," p. 1733.

7. The National Cholesterol Education Program created a Laboratory Standards Committee to consider the problem of inaccurate total blood cholesterol tests. The committee published its standards in 1988, proposing provisional standards that became progressively more stringent each year until the committee's final standards were reached in 1992. See James O. Westgard, Per Hyltoft Petersen, and Donald A. Wiebe, "Laboratory Process Specifications for Assuring Quality in the U.S. National Cholesterol Education Program," *Clinical Chemistry* 37, no. 5 (1991): 656–61. The standards are voluntary.

8. IARC Working Group on Evaluation of Cervical Cancer Screening Programmes, "Screening for Squamous Cervical Cancer: Duration of Low Risk after Negative Results of Cervical Cytology and Its Implications for Screening Policies,"

British Medical Journal 293 (September 13, 1986): Table 1 and p. 661; see also Anthony B. Miller, "Screening for Cancer: State of the Art and Prospects for the Future," *World Journal of Surgery* 131 (January–February 1989): 79–83.

9. These estimates of cost-effectiveness do not come from the same studies as the estimates of annual costs presented above. In general, they are somewhat more complete than the annual estimates, but it is not possible to derive annual estimates from them.

10. Lee Goldman, Milton C. Weinstein, Paula A. Goldman, and Lawrence W. Williams, "Cost-Effectiveness of HMG-CoA Reductase Inhibition for Primary and Secondary Prevention of Coronary Heart Disease," *Journal of the American Medical Association* 265 (March 6, 1991): 1145.

11. Jan-Erik Johansson, Hans-Olov Adami, Swen-Olof Andersson, Reinhold Bergstrom, Lars Holmberg, and Ulla Brith Krusemo, "High 10-Year Survival Rate in Patients with Early, Untreated Prostatic Cancer," *Journal of the American Medical Association* 267 (April 22/29, 1992): 2191–96.

12. See the appendix to Chapter 5 for details on the derivation of the estimates presented in Figure 5.

13. Marilyn J. Field and Kathleen N. Lohr, eds., *Guidelines for Clinical Practice: From Development to Use (Summary)* (Washington, D.C.: National Academy Press, 1992), p. 10.

14. Field and Lohr, *Guidelines for Clinical Practice*, p. 8.

15. U.S. Preventive Services Task Force, *Guide to Clinical Preventive Services: An Assessment of the Effectiveness of 169 Interventions* (Baltimore: Williams and Wilkins, 1989), appendix A.

16. Two of its reports have been important sources for this monograph: Charlotte Muller, Jeanne Mandelblatt, Clyde B. Shechter, Elaine J. Power, Brigitte M. Duffy, and Judith L. Wagner, *The Costs and Effectiveness of Cervical Cancer Screening in Elderly Women* (Office of Technology Assess-

ment, U.S. Congress, February 1990); and Alan M. Garber, Benjamin Littenberg, Harold C. Sox, Jr., Michael E. Gluck, Judith L. Wagner, and Brigitte M. Duffy, *Costs and Effectiveness of Cholesterol Screening in the Elderly* (Office of Technology Assessment, U.S. Congress, April 1989).

17. See David M. Eddy in the preface to David M. Eddy, ed., *Common Screening Tests* (Philadelphia: American College of Physicians, 1991).

18. Louise B. Russell, "Proposed: A Comprehensive Health Care System for the Poor," *The Brookings Review* 7 (Summer 1989): 13–20.

19. David C. Hadorn, "Setting Health Care Priorities in Oregon: Cost-Effectiveness Meets the Rule of Rescue," *Journal of the American Medical Association* 265 (May 1, 1991): 2218–225.

20. Patrick Walsh is quoted in Ron Winslow, "Test Changes Prostate Cancer Treatment," *Wall Street Journal*, April 22, 1992, pp. B1ff.

Index

Compositor: ComCom, Inc.
       Text: 10/14 Aster
    Display: Aster
    Printer: Haddon Craftsmen, Inc.
     Binder: Haddon Craftsmen, Inc.